Covid-19 Airway Management and Ventilation Strategy for Critically Ill Older Patients

Nicola Vargas · Antonio M. Esquinas
Editors

Covid-19 Airway Management and Ventilation Strategy for Critically Ill Older Patients

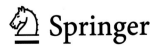 Springer

Editors
Nicola Vargas
Geriatric and Intensive Geriatric Cares
San Giuseppe Moscati Hospital
Avellino
Italy

Antonio M. Esquinas
International NIV School
and Fellow Program
Intensive Care Unit
Hospital Morales Meseguer
Murcia
Spain

ISBN 978-3-030-55623-5   ISBN 978-3-030-55621-1   (eBook)
https://doi.org/10.1007/978-3-030-55621-1

This Springer imprint is published by the registered company Springer Nature Switzerland AG
The registered company address is: Gewerbestrasse 11, 6330 Cham, Switzerland

Preface

Older adults are more susceptible to complications such as acute respiratory distress syndrome (ARDS) as a result of COVID-19 viral pneumonia. They are commonly frail and with multiple comorbidities. Frailty means reduced functional reserve of the different organs and systems such as the respiratory system. Hence, older adults have less ability to react to acute stressors. During the current COVID-19 pandemic, older adult patients' mortality is increased. The contagious and death rate of elderly in nursing homes and health care residences is high. Older adults with COVID disease management is complicated. The reduced availability of ICU beds may limit their access to ICU. On the other hand, the prognosis may be weak, and the airway management and ventilation strategy must take into account many specific elder clinic and physiologic characteristics.

Avellino, Italy   Nicola Vargas
Murcia, Spain   Antonio M. Esquinas

Contents

Part I

Epidemiology

Mortality and Prognosis of Older Patients During COVID-19 Pandemic

Sonia Alvarado de la Torre, Manuel Ángel Gómez-Ríos, and Zeping Xu

1.1 Epidemiological Perspective: A Global View of the Problem

An ongoing outbreak of pneumonia caused by the severe acute respiratory coronavirus 2 (SARS-CoV-2) started in December 2009 in Wuhan, China, and was gradually spread around the world. This is the third coronavirus infection in two decades, after the severe acute respiratory syndrome (SARS) and the Middle East respiratory syndrome (MERS). It was officially named Corona Virus Disease 2019 (COVID-19) by the World Health Organization (WHO), in February 2020. Since then, the virus has become widespread, turning into a pandemic, in March 2020. Currently, the number of people diagnosed with COVID-19 worldwide has crossed the five million mark, causing more than 300,000 deaths.

The scientific community offered the first clinical reports according to the disease has been spread, mainly case series from mainland China. These publications provided the first descriptions of clinical, pathological, and epidemiological characteristics of the disease. In all of them, including others published afterward from worldwide, many epidemiological characteristics have become constant. Thus, the majority of the infected population is over 50 years, while the majority of the deceased are alder than 60 years [1]. Disease severity and death are associated with elderly and age-related comorbidity [1, 2]. The median age of the deceased was 80 years (interquartile range, 30–103) in Italy; only 1.1% of those who died were aged less than 50 years; 51.2% of patients who died had three or more age-related

S. A. de la Torre · M. Á. Gómez-Ríos (✉)
Department of Anesthesiology and Perioperative Medicine, University Hospital Complex of A Coruña, A Coruña, Spain

Z. Xu
Department of Anesthesiology, Jiangsu Cancer Hospital, Nanjing, China

© The Editor(s) (if applicable) and The Author(s), under exclusive license to Springer Nature Switzerland AG 2020
N. Vargas, A. M. Esquinas (eds.), *Covid-19 Airway Management and Ventilation Strategy for Critically Ill Older Patients*, https://doi.org/10.1007/978-3-030-55621-1_1

diseases, such as cardiac ischemia, hypertension, type II diabetes mellitus, and chronic obstructive pulmonary disease [2]. Young et al. [3] found pre-existing comorbidities were associated with a CFR of 10.5% (cardiovascular disease), 7.3% (diabetes), 6.3% (chronic respiratory disease), 6.0% (hypertension), and 5.6% (cancer). Severe COVID-19 forms include acute respiratory distress syndrome (ARDS), hyper-inflammatory syndrome, thromboembolic disorders, acute kidney injury [4, 5], and liver dysfunction, and multi-organ failure. Wu et al. [6] studied the risk factors of evolution to ARDS and death in patients with COVID-19 in Wuhan, in a sample of 201 hospitalized patients. They found that older age (≥65 years) was associated with a higher risk of ARDS (HR 3.26, 95% CI 2.08–5.11) and death (HR 6.17; 95% CI 3.26–11.67). Likewise, Zhou et al. [7] in a retrospective cohort study of 191 patients found that older age (≥60) was an independent risk factor for mortality of adult inpatients with COVID-19. Mo et al. [8] analyzed the clinical characteristic associated with what they called "Refractory COVID-19 pneumonia" (no clinical or radiological remission within 10 days of hospitalization). Elderly age was the main risk factor for developing refractory COVID-19 pneumonia and was associated with higher in-hospital mortality rate. Figure 1.1 shows pre-existing comorbidities associate with high case fatality rate.

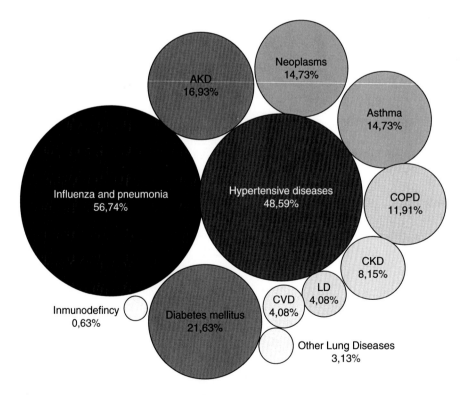

Fig. 1.1 Common comorbidities in COVID-19 patients. *AKD* acute kidney disease, *CKD* chronic kidney disease, *LD* liver diseases, *CVD* cardiovascular disease. (Image adapted from Hasan Z, Narasimhan M. Preparing for the COVID-19 Pandemic: Our Experience in New York. Chest 2020 [9])

These initial findings were contrasted by Verity et al. [10]. They estimated the severity of COVID-19 in mainland China using a model-based analysis collecting clinical information of 70,117 patients. The authors estimated a case fatality ratio of 1.38% in China, with substantially higher ratios in elderly age groups (0.32% in those aged <60 years; 4.5% in those aged ≥60 years; and up to 13.4% in those aged 80 years and older). These findings were later confirmed in Lombardy, Italy, one of the most affected European countries. Grasselli et al. [11] noted that older patients ≥64 years admitted to ICUs had higher mortality than patients <64 years (36% vs. 15%). Kang et al. [12] found an overall death rate of 1% in a population of Korea while the mortality rate leaped to 5.2% for patients in their 70s and 9.2% in their 80s. Richardson et al. [13] published a case series of 5700 hospitalized patients in New York obtaining similar results. Table 1.1 shows the association between old age and mortality risk.

Many elderly patients stay at home or live in a Long-Term Care Facility without being admitted to hospital, especially in developed countries with aging populations. Data from these population subgroups are less frequent. McMichael et al. [14] evaluated the epidemiological characteristics of COVID-19 in a Long-Term Care Facility in Washington. They found a case fatality rate of 33.7%. These results cannot be extrapolated to the general population, but warn of a larger problem.

Currently, available evidence indicates that COVID-19 is a "gerolavic infection" (from Greek, géros "old man," and epilavís "harmful") taking into account these features constantly present regardless of studied country, its rent per capita or the characteristics of their health systems. It disproportionately affects the elderly. Nevertheless, consider old age in isolation as a risk factor is an oversimplified view of the matter, since the presence of comorbidity, especially cardiovascular diseases (mainly hypertension), diabetes, and chronic lung diseases, were constantly associated with the worst prognosis. All these diseases are common in older patients, and even are strongly related to the aging process. In fact, many of the COVID-19 patients over 65 years have at least one comorbidity of them. Therefore, it is difficult to attribute the higher incidence of death to one independent risk factor. In addition, there is still scarce of accurate statistics linking smoking, lifestyle, and behavior to the severity and lethality of COVID-19 [15, 16]. Table 1.2 shows the different comorbidity and risk of suffering severe forms of the disease.

Table 1.1 Older age and risk of mortality

Study	Country	Sample	Age (years)	Mortality HR (95%CI)	p-value
Wu et al. [6]	China	201	>65	3.26 (2.08–5.11)	<0.001
Zhou et al. [7]	China	191	>60	1.1 (1.03–1017, per year increase)	0.0043
Verity et al. [10]	China	70,177	≥60	4.5 (1.18–11.10)	<0.001
Grasselli et al. [11]	Italy	1591	≥64	2.1 (1.70–2.60)[a]	<0.001
Kang et al. [12]	Korea	8236	>70 >80	3.84 6.71	
Richardson et al. [13]	USA	5700	>65	3.12	

[a]Mortality in the intensive care unit

Table 1.2 Comorbidity and risk of severe forms of COVID-19

Study	Country	Sample	Comorbidity	HR (95%CI)	*p*-value
Chen et al. [17]	China	1590	>75 years Coronary heart disease Cerebrovascular disease	7.86 (2.44–25.35) 4.28 (1.14–16.11) 3.1 (1.07–8.94)	<0.01
Zhang et al. [18]	China	663	>60 years Chronic diseases		<0.001 <0.001
Zhu et al. [19]	China	127	Hypertension	4.38 (1.01–18.99)	<0.05
Liu et al. [20]	China	99	Hypertension >65 years	3.59 (1.01–12.58) 1.85 (0.52–6.41)	0.048 0.347
Du et al. [21]	China	179	≥65 years Hypertension Cardiovascular/ cerebrovascular disease	9.74 (3.11–30.06) 4.08 (1.58–10.51) 11.05 (4.06–30.06)	<0.001 0.004 <0.001
Wang et al. [22]	China	1558	Hypertension Diabetes COPD[a] Cardiovascular disease Cerebrovascular disease	2.29 (1.69–3.10) 2.47 (1.67–3.66) 5.97 (2.49–14.29) 2.93 (1.73–4.96) 3.89 (1.64–9.22)	<0.001 <0.001 <0.001 <0.001 <0.001
Zhang et al. [23]	China	111	Male gender >1 Comorbidity[b]	24.8 (1.8–342.1) 52.6 (3.6–776.4)	0.016 0.004
Yu et al. [24]	China	95	≥65 years High BMI[c]	1.03 (1.01–1.05) 1.14 (0.99–1.32)	0.025 0.057
Zheng et al. [25]	China	3027	Male Gender >65 years Smoking Hypertension Diabetes Cardiovascular disease COPD	1.76 (1.41–2.18) 6.06 (3.98–9.22) 2.51 (1.39–3.32) 2.72 (1.60–4.64) 3.68 (2.68–5.03) 5.19 (3.25–8.29) 5.15 (2.51–10.57)	<0.001 <0.001 <0.001 <0.001 <0.001 <0.001 <0.001
Li et al. [26] (32294485)	China	549	≥65 years Hypertension	2.2 (1.5–3.5) 2 (1.3–3.2)	<0.001 <0.001
Chen et al. [17]	China	1590	≥75 years 65–74 years Coronary heart disease Cerebrovascular disease	7.86 (2.44–25.35) 3.43 (1.24–9.5) 4.28 (1.14–16.13) 3.1 (1.07–8.94)	<0.001 <0.001 <0.001 <0.001
Wei et al. [27]	China	167	Comorbidity >65 years	3.12 (1.3–7.11) 1.038 (1.009–1.68)	0.007 0.009

[a]*COPD* chronic obstructive pulmonary disease
[b]Comorbidities (hypertension, diabetes, chronic obstructive pulmonary disease, malignancy, cancer and chronic liver disease)
[c]*BMI* body mass index

1.2 Why the Elderly Is at Higher Risk? A Pathophysiological View

The relationship between older age and COVID-19 disease deserves an analysis of the causes that could justify these findings. Two aspects must be considered: the pathogen agent and host–virus interaction.

COVID-19 is an infectious disease caused by SARS-CoV-2, an enveloped, positive-sense, single-stranded RNA virus of high infectivity [28]. Routes of viral transmission include respiratory droplets, aerosolization, and possible direct contact. It is plausible that SARS-CoV-2 could cause infection through close eye contact or fecal–oral route [29, 30]. The reproductive number of SARS-CoV-2 (number of people infected from one infected person) is around 2.68 [31]. The virus can trigger a violent dysregulated immune host response mediated by a "cytokine storm" released by immune effector cells that can result in severe outcomes in most of these older patients as ARDS, multiple organ failure, and death [32].

The SARS-Cov-2 penetrates into host cells via angiotensin-converting-enzyme-2 (ACE2) receptors, and viral RNA enters the nucleus for replication. ACE2 is ubiquitous and widely expressed in the heart, vascular endothelium, gut, lung (particularly in type 2 pneumocytes and macrophages), kidney, bladder, and brain [33–35]. Therefore, these organs could be more vulnerable [32] explaining the wide variety of clinical manifestations of the disease [36–38].

SARS-CoV2 downregulates ACE2 receptors mediated by increased activity of ADAM metallopeptidase domain 17 (ADAM17), which cleaves ACE2 from the cell membrane. Thus, its catalytic effect of angiotensin II (among its effects: vasoconstriction, enhanced inflammation, and thrombosis) to angiotensin1–7 (counter-regulatory protective effects: vasodilatory, anti-inflammatory, antifibrotic, and antigrowth effects) is lost, while pro-inflammatory cytokines are released into the circulation [39]. Both phenomena can destabilize a pre-existing pulmonary, cardiovascular, or kidney illness, or result in the loss of homeostasis of an organ/system with limited functional reserve [40]. Several entities associated with infection and severity of the disease as older age, hypertension, diabetes, and cardiovascular disease share an ACE2 deficiency. Verdecchia et al. [34] suggest that ACE2 downregulation induced by SARS-CoV2 might cause a hyper-inflammatory reaction being especially detrimental in people with baseline ACE2 deficiency since it might amplify the dysregulation of angiotensin II–angiotensin1–7. This dysregulation could result in abundant neutrophil infiltration, and progression of severe pulmonary inflammatory and thrombotic processes [4]. Likewise, ACE2 may be upregulated in patients with cardiac disease and treated with ACE inhibitors or angiotensin receptor blockers. ACE2 upregulation may increase the susceptibility to COVID-19 but might be also protective versus angiotensin II mediated vasoconstriction and inflammatory activation [40]. There are lack of untoward effects of ACE inhibitors or angiotensin receptor blockers for COVID-19 infection and severity. The American Heart Association and the European Society of Cardiology recommend that these antihypertensive drugs should not be discontinued until more evidence is available [5, 41–43].

On the other hand, it is necessary to evaluate the role of senescence in the pathophysiology of COVID-19 [44]. The aging process is characterized by the gradual development of a chronic subclinical systemic inflammation (inflamm-aging) and by progressive immune system impairment (immune senescence) that cause the progressive deterioration of the organ systems function promoting the appearance of age-related diseases, cognitive decline, dependency, and, therefore, frailty [45]. The progressive loss of physiological functional reserve leads to a state of vulnerability. The rate of inflamm-aging is higher in men. This fact agrees that male gender could be a risk factor for adverse outcomes of the disease [46].

Macrophages are recruited by SARS-CoV-2-infected cells expressing ACE2. Senescent-like macrophages compound the inflammation induced by COVID-19 through the production of pro-inflammatory cytokines like IL-6 [2]. Likewise, IL-6 elevation is typical of aging and chronic disease [47]. Persistent IL-6 elevation can promote lung tissue inflammation and injury and viral replication [48, 49]. Targeting IL-6 attenuates the cytokine storm [50]. Tociluzimab is an immunoregolatory drug used to treat rheumatoid artritis and can have some efficacy against the effects of systemic IL-6 elevation in COVID-19 infection [51]. Acute SARS-Cov-2 infection compounds the chronic pro-inflammatory state which, together with immune senescence and the age-specific distribution of ACE2 in the airway epithelia, could blunt the antiviral response to inflammation. This model could explain the delayed viral clearance and the high rate of adverse outcomes in older patients [2]. In older patient with the highest rate of inflamm-aging, the inflammatory response induced by SARS-Cov-2 infection seems to favor a poorer outcome [2].

Bonafè et al. [2] hypothesize that in addition to the downregulation of ACE2 several aging-related features could explain why the elderly suffers a severe disease with high mortality as the presence of subclinical systemic inflammation; a basal blunted immune system and type I interferon response due to the chronic inflammation; and accelerated biological aging, as measured by epigenetic and senescence markers (e.g., telomere shortening) associated to the chronic inflammatory state.

NICE guidelines recommend that a fragility assessment be carried out for all patients using the Clinical Frailty Score (CFS) [52]. Frailty scores are a useful tool in making decisions. The CFS considers age, functional baseline, and comorbid conditions, grading patients from 1 (very fit) to 9 (terminally ill). Patients with a CFS score less than 5 (slightly fragile) could benefit to a greater extent from organ support treatment in critical care [32]. Many of the frail score items constitute risk factors of death in patients with COVID-19. All of them are related to the aging process. Therefore, senescence, comorbidity, and frailty are different but closely related concepts that play a role in the pathogenic mechanism of COVID-19 disease [53].

1.3 Prognosis of the COVID-19 Elderly Patient

Currently, there is scarce evidence on long-term prognosis or quality of life of recovered elderly patients. Recent research focuses on evaluating the short-term related outcomes (death, progression of disease severity, discharge from hospital, or viral clearance studies) after infection is diagnosed (see Table 1.3) [59]. In this regard, it is important to bear in mind that the elderly population may present atypically with delirium, postural instability, or diarrhea, and without typical respiratory symptoms and fever [1]. Several retrospective cohort studies examined the prognostic ability of one or more baseline factors to predict subsequent evolution. This information could support decision-making to provide appropriate individualized

Table 1.3 Characteristics and studied outcomes of different short-term prognostic studies

References	Sample Size	Hospital	Outcomes
Guan et al. [54]	1590	575 Hospitals across China, nationwide	ICU admission, invasive ventilation, mortality
Chen et al. [55]	701 (442 included in prognostic analysis)	Tongji Hospital, Wuhan, China	Mortality, association between kidney disease and in-hospital death
Chen et al. [56]	249	Shanghai Publical Health Clinical Center, Shanghai, China	ICU admission, mortality
Cai et al. [57]	298	Third people's Hospital of Shenzhen, Guangdong, China	Mortality
Gao et al. [58]	54	Union Hospital of Huazhong University of Science and Technology, Wuhan, China	Mortality

treatment and optimizing the use of medical resources at a time when they are urgently needed.

All the research showed the association between increasing age and worse prognosis [1]. Death rate could be more than double in the over 65s [55]. In addition to age, male gender, and presence of comorbidity (body mass index, hypertension, diabetes, COPD, coronary heart disease, and malignant tumors), specific laboratory and radiology findings are important prognostic factors [1]. Patients with two or more comorbidities have a poorer prognosis than patients with one [60]. Higher levels of fever and higher respiratory rate are associated with increased rates of progression or mortality. Higher levels of procalcitonin, high-sensitivity C-reactive protein, IL-6, D-dimer, myoglobin, high-sensitivity cardiac troponin I, white blood cell counts, creatinine, urea, creatine kinase, lactate dehydrogenase, total bilirubin and lower lymphocyte counts and albumin are consistently associated with worse prognosis [1, 7, 61]. Severe disease was associated with a cytokine storm, fundamentally higher levels of circulating IL-6 [62, 63]. A strong association between the presence of fewer lymphocytes, more neutrophils, and higher neutrophil-to-lymphocyte ratio level (NLR) and the severity of COVID-19 have also been identified [64–67].

Different set of predictors have been described. Bai et al. [68] identified age >55 years, hypertension, decreased albumin, decreased lymphocyte count, elevated CRP, progressive consolidation, and lack of fibrosis at initial CT scan as associated with higher risk of progression to severe disease. Yan et al. [69] identified higher lactic dehydrogenase, lower lymphocytes, and higher high-sensitivity CRP as associated with greater risk of mortality. However, proposed models could be poorly reported, at high risk of bias [70].

Ji et al. [71] described the first prediction progression score called "CALL Score." It includes comorbidity (hypertension, diabetes, cardiovascular diseases, pulmonary and cerebrovascular disease), older age (more than 60 years old), lower lymphocyte, and higher lactate dehydrogenase at presentation were independent high-risk factors for COVID-19. The score achieved a good concordance index of 0.86, and its area under the ROC curve was 0.91 (95% CI, 0.86–0.94). Furthermore, CALL Score was classified into three levels of risk according to the probability of progression. Those with 4–6 points had less than 10% probabilities to progression and were considered low-risk patients; 7–9 points with 10–40% probabilities of progression were intermediate-risk; and 10–13 points with over 40% probabilities were high-risk. This score is a practical tool but it needs to be validated with a large prospective multicenter study. Similarly, Liang et al. [72] developed the COVID risk score based on ten variables (X-ray abnormality, age, hemoptysis, dyspnea, unconsciousness, number of comorbidities, cancer history, NLR, lactate dehydrogenase, and direct bilirubin) commonly measured on admission to the hospital.

Previous validated critical ill scores (Acute Physiology and Chronic Health Evaluation II score (APACHE II score), the Sequential Organ Failure Assessment score (SOFA score), and the Confusion, Urea, Respiratory rate, Blood pressure, Age 65 score "CURB65 score") can also be useful in decision-making. Interestingly, both APACHE II and CURB65 included older age as poor prognosis factors. Zou et al. [73] had studied which of them was more effective to predict hospital mortality in patients with COVID-19. APACHE II was identified as the most efficient with an area under ROC curve of 0.966. They also concluded that an APACHE II score greater than or equal to 17 serves as an early-warning indicator of death and may provide a useful guidance.

The assessment of biological and immunological aging markers as frailty scores and composite inflammatory could be a valuable strategy for COVID-19 patient risk stratification [2].

Several studies suggest that the ongoing active alveolitis during the host immune system response might lead to pulmonary fibrosis after recovery in some patients [74]. In addition, they may have suffered isolation and its long-term consequences as anxiety, depression, or neurocognitive disorders [1, 36].

References

1. Lithander FE, Neumann S, Tenison E, Lloyd K, Welsh TJ, Rodrigues JCL, Higgins JPT, Scourfield L, Christensen H, Haunton VJ, et al. COVID-19 in older people: a rapid clinical review. Age Ageing. 2020;49:501–15.
2. Bonafè M, Prattichizzo F, Giuliani A, Storci G, Sabbatinelli J, Olivieri F. Inflamm-aging: why older men are the most susceptible to SARS-CoV-2 complicated outcomes. Cytokine Growth Factor Rev. 2020;53:33.
3. Young BE, Ong SWX, Kalimuddin S, Low JG, Tan SY, Loh J, Ng OT, Marimuthu K, Ang LW, Mak TM, et al. Epidemiologic features and clinical course of patients infected with SARS-CoV-2 in Singapore. JAMA. 2020;323:1488–94.
4. Connors JM, Levy JH. COVID-19 and its implications for thrombosis and anticoagulation. Blood. 2020;135:2033.
5. Mehra MR, Desai SS, Kuy S, Henry TD, Patel AN. Cardiovascular disease, drug therapy, and mortality in Covid-19. N Engl J Med. 2020;382:2582.

6. Wu C, Chen X, Cai Y, Xia J, Zhou X, Xu S, Huang H, Zhang L, Du C, Zhang Y, et al. Risk factors associated with acute respiratory distress syndrome and death in patients with coronavirus disease 2019 Pneumonia in Wuhan, China. JAMA Intern Med. 2020. https://doi.org/10.1001/jamainternmed.2020.0994.

7. Zhou F, Yu T, Du R, Fan G, Liu Y, Liu Z, Xiang J, Wang Y, Song B, Gu X, et al. Clinical course and risk factors for mortality of adult inpatients with COVID-19 in Wuhan, China: a retrospective cohort study. Lancet. 2020;395(10229):1054–62.

8. Mo P, Xing Y, Xiao Y, Deng L, Zhao Q, Wang H, Xiong Y, Cheng Z, Gao S, Liang K, et al. Clinical characteristics of refractory COVID-19 pneumonia in Wuhan, China. Clin Infect Dis. 2020;2020:ciaa270.

9. Hasan Z, Narasimhan M. Preparing for the COVID-19 pandemic: our experience in New York. Chest. 2020;157:1420.

10. Verity R, Okell LC, Dorigatti I, Winskill P, Whittaker C, Imai N, Cuomo-Dannenburg G, Thompson H, Walker PGT, Fu H, et al. Estimates of the severity of coronavirus disease 2019: a model-based analysis. Lancet Infect Dis. 2020;20:669–77.

11. Grasselli G, Zangrillo A, Zanella A, Antonelli M, Cabrini L, Castelli A, Cereda D, Coluccello A, Foti G, Fumagalli R, et al. Baseline characteristics and outcomes of 1591 patients infected with SARS-CoV-2 admitted to ICUs of the Lombardy Region, Italy. JAMA. 2020;323:1574–81.

12. Kang YJ. Mortality rate of infection with COVID-19 in Korea from the perspective of underlying disease. Disaster Med Public Health Prep. 2020:1–3.

13. Richardson S, Hirsch JS, Narasimhan M, Crawford JM, McGinn T, Davidson KW, Barnaby DP, Becker LB, Chelico JD, Cohen SL, et al. Presenting characteristics, comorbidities, and outcomes among 5700 patients hospitalized with COVID-19 in the New York City Area. JAMA. 2020;323:2052–9.

14. McMichael TM, Currie DW, Clark S, Pogosjans S, Kay M, Schwartz NG, Lewis J, Baer A, Kawakami V, Lukoff MD, et al. Epidemiology of Covid-19 in a long-term care facility in King County, Washington. N Engl J Med. 2020;382:2005–11.

15. Zhavoronkov A. Geroprotective and senoremediative strategies to reduce the comorbidity, infection rates, severity, and lethality in gerophilic and gerolavic infections. Aging (Albany NY). 2020;12(8):6492–510.

16. Hefler M, Gartner CE. The tobacco industry in the time of COVID-19: time to shut it down? Tob Control. 2020;29:245–6.

17. Chen R, Liang W, Jiang M, et al. Risk Factors of Fatal Outcome in Hospitalized Subjects With Coronavirus Disease 2019 From a Nationwide Analysis in China. Chest. 2020;158(1):97–105. https://doi.org/10.1016/j.chest.2020.04.010.

18. Zhang J, Wang X, Jia X, et al. Risk factors for disease severity, unimprovement, and mortality in COVID-19 patients in Wuhan, China. Clin Microbiol Infect. 2020;26(6):767–72. https://doi.org/10.1016/j.cmi.2020.04.012.

19. Zhu Z, Cai T, Fan L, Lou K, Hua X, Huang Z, Gao G. Clinical value of immune-inflammatory parameters to assess the severity of coronavirus disease 2019. Int J Infect Dis. 2020;95:332–9.

20. Liu X, Zhou H, Zhou Y, et al. Risk factors associated with disease severity and length of hospital stay in COVID-19 patients. J Infect. 2020;81(1):e95–e97. https://doi.org/10.1016/j.jinf.2020.04.008.

21. Du RH, Liang LR, Yang CQ, Wang W, Cao TZ, Li M, Guo GY, Du J, Zheng CL, Zhu Q, et al. Predictors of mortality for patients with COVID-19 pneumonia caused by SARS-CoV-2: a prospective cohort study. Eur Respir J. 2020;55:5.

22. Wang B, Li R, Lu Z, Huang Y. Does comorbidity increase the risk of patients with COVID-19: evidence from meta-analysis. Aging (Albany NY). 2020;12(7):6049–57.

23. Zhang J, Yu M, Tong S, Liu LY, Tang LV. Predictive factors for disease progression in hospitalized patients with coronavirus disease 2019 in Wuhan, China. J Clin Virol. 2020;127:104392.

24. Yu T, Cai S, Zheng Z, Cai X, Liu Y, Yin S, Peng J, Xu X. Association between clinical manifestations and prognosis in patients with COVID-19. Clin Ther. 2020;42:964.

25. Zheng Z, Peng F, Xu B, et al. Risk factors of critical & mortal COVID-19 cases: A systematic literature review and meta-analysis. J Infect. 2020;81(2):e16–e25. https://doi.org/10.1016/j.jinf.2020.04.021.

26. Li X, Xu S, Yu M, et al. Risk factors for severity and mortality in adult COVID-19 inpatients in Wuhan. J Allergy Clin Immunol. 2020;146(1):110–18. https://doi.org/10.1016/j.jaci.2020.04.006.

27. Wei YY, Wang RR, Zhang DW, et al. Risk factors for severe COVID-19: Evidence from 167 hospitalized patients in Anhui, China [published online ahead of print, 2020 Apr 17]. J Infect. 2020. https://doi.org/10.1016/j.jinf.2020.04.010.

28. Yuki K, Fujiogi M, Koutsogiannaki S. COVID-19 pathophysiology: a review. Clin Immunol. 2020;215:108427.

29. Tang LY, Wang J. Anesthesia and COVID-19: what we should know and what we should do. Semin Cardiothorac Vasc Anesth. 2020;24(2):127–37.

30. Yeo C, Kaushal S, Yeo D. Enteric involvement of coronaviruses: is faecal-oral transmission of SARS-CoV-2 possible? Lancet Gastroenterol Hepatol. 2020;5(4):335–7.

31. Wu JT, Leung K, Leung GM. Nowcasting and forecasting the potential domestic and international spread of the 2019-nCoV outbreak originating in Wuhan, China: a modelling study. Lancet. 2020;395(10225):689–97.

32. Down B, Kulkarni S, Ahmed Khan AH, Barker B, Tang I. Novel coronavirus (COVID-19) infection: what a doctor on the frontline needs to know. Ann Med Surg (Lond). 2020;55:24.

33. Wong CK, Lam CW, Wu AK, Ip WK, Lee NL, Chan IH, Lit LC, Hui DS, Chan MH, Chung SS. Plasma inflammatory cytokines and chemokines in severe acute respiratory syndrome. Clin Exp Immunol. 2004;136(1):95–103.

34. Verdecchia P, Cavallini C, Spanevello A, Angeli F. The pivotal link between ACE2 deficiency and SARS-CoV-2 infection. Eur J Intern Med. 2020;76:14.

35. Varga Z, Flammer AJ, Steiger P, Haberecker M, Andermatt R, Zinkernagel AS, Mehra MR, Schuepbach RA, Ruschitzka F, Moch H. Endothelial cell infection and endotheliitis in COVID-19. Lancet. 2020;395(10234):1417–8.

36. Balachandar V, Mahalaxmi I, Subramaniam M, Kaavya J, Senthil Kumar N, Laldinmawii G, Narayanasamy A, Janardhana Kumar Reddy P, Sivaprakash P, Kanchana S, et al. Follow-up studies in COVID-19 recovered patients—is it mandatory? Sci Total Environ. 2020;729:139021.

37. Klonoff DC, Umpierrez GE. COVID-19 in patients with diabetes: risk factors that increase morbidity. Metabolism. 2020;108:154224.

38. Long B, Brady WJ, Koyfman A, Gottlieb M. Cardiovascular complications in COVID-19. Am J Emerg Med. 2020;38:1504.

39. Tay MZ, Poh CM, Rénia L, MacAry PA, Ng LFP. The trinity of COVID-19: immunity, inflammation and intervention. Nat Rev Immunol. 2020;20:363.

40. Tomasoni D, Italia L, Adamo M, et al. COVID-19 and heart failure: from infection to inflammation and angiotensin II stimulation. Searching for evidence from a new disease [published online ahead of print, 2020 May 15]. Eur J Heart Fail. 2020; https://doi.org/10.1002/ejhf.1871.

41. Rossi GP, Sanga V, Barton M. Potential harmful effects of discontinuing ACE-inhibitors and ARBs in COVID-19 patients. elife. 2020;9:e57278.

42. Rico-Mesa JS, White A, Anderson AS. Outcomes in patients with COVID-19 infection taking ACEI/ARB. Curr Cardiol Rep. 2020;22(5):31.

43. Talreja H, Tan J, Dawes M, Supershad S, Rabindranath K, Fisher J, Valappil S, van der Merwe V, Wong L, van der Merwe W, et al. A consensus statement on the use of angiotensin receptor blockers and angiotensin converting enzyme inhibitors in relation to COVID-19 (corona virus disease 2019). N Z Med J. 2020;133(1512):85–7.

44. Lauc G, Sinclair D. Biomarkers of biological age as predictors of COVID-19 disease severity. Aging (Albany NY). 2020;12(8):6490–1.

45. Gomez-Rios MA, Casans-Frances R, Abad-Gurumeta A. Improving perioperative outcomes in the frail elderly patient. Minerva Anestesiol. 2019;85:1154–6.

46. Liu K, Chen Y, Lin R, Han K. Clinical features of COVID-19 in elderly patients: a comparison with young and middle-aged patients. J Inf Secur. 2020;80(6):e14–8.

47. Maggio M, Guralnik JM, Longo DL, Ferrucci L. Interleukin-6 in aging and chronic disease: a magnificent pathway. J Gerontol A Biol Sci Med Sci. 2006;61(6):575–84.

48. Yu M, Zheng X, Witschi H, Pinkerton KE. The role of interleukin-6 in pulmonary inflammation and injury induced by exposure to environmental air pollutants. Toxicol Sci. 2002;68(2):488–97.
49. Velazquez-Salinas L, Verdugo-Rodriguez A, Rodriguez LL, Borca MV. The role of interleukin 6 during viral infections. Front Microbiol. 2019;10:1057.
50. Lee DW, Gardner R, Porter DL, Louis CU, Ahmed N, Jensen M, Grupp SA, Mackall CL. Current concepts in the diagnosis and management of cytokine release syndrome. Blood. 2014;124(2):188–95.
51. Cytokine Storm Drugs Move from CAR T to COVID-19. Cancer Discov. 2020;10(7):OF8. https://doi.org/10.1158/2159-8290. CD-ND2020-008.
52. Available at COVID-19 rapid guideline: managing suspected or confirmed pneumonia in adults in the community NICE guideline [NG165]. https://www.nice.org.uk/guidance/ng165.
53. Makary MA, Segev DL, Pronovost PJ, Syin D, Bandeen-Roche K, Patel P, Takenaga R, Devgan L, Holzmueller CG, Tian J, et al. Frailty as a predictor of surgical outcomes in older patients. J Am Coll Surg. 2010;210(6):901–8.
54. Guan WJ, Liang WH, Zhao Y, et al. Comorbidity and its impact on 1590 patients with COVID-19 in China: a nationwide analysis. Eur Respir J. 2020;55(5):2000547. Published 2020 May 14. https://doi.org/10.1183/13993003.00547-2020.
55. Cheng Y, Luo R, Wang K, Zhang M, Wang Z, Dong L, Li J, Yao Y, Ge S, Xu G. Kidney disease is associated with in-hospital death of patients with COVID-19. Kidney Int. 2020;97(5):829–38.
56. Chen J, Qi T, Liu L, Ling Y, Qian Z, Li T, Li F, Xu Q, Zhang Y, Xu S, et al. Clinical progression of patients with COVID-19 in Shanghai, China. J Inf Secur. 2020;80(5):e1–6.
57. Cai Q, Huang D, Ou P, et al. COVID-19 in a designated infectious diseases hospital outside Hubei Province, China. Allergy. 2020;75(7):1742–52. https://doi.org/10.1111/all.14309.
58. Gao L, Jiang D, Wen XS, Cheng XC, Sun M, He B, You LN, Lei P, Tan XW, Qin S, et al. Prognostic value of NT-nBNP in patients with severe COVID-19. Respir Res. 2020;21(1):83.
59. Sun Y, Koh V, Marimuthu K, et al. Epidemiological and Clinical Predictors of COVID-19. Clin Infect Dis. 2020;71(15):786–92. https://doi.org/10.1093/cid/ciaa322.
60. Guan WJ, Ni ZY, Hu Y, Liang WH, Ou CQ, He JX, Liu L, Shan H, Lei CL, Hui DSC, et al. Clinical characteristics of coronavirus disease 2019 in China. N Engl J Med. 2020;382(18):1708–20.
61. Ruan Q, Yang K, Wang W, Jiang L, Song J. Clinical predictors of mortality due to COVID-19 based on an analysis of data of 150 patients from Wuhan, China. Intens Care Med. 2020;46(5):846–8.
62. Huang C, Wang Y, Li X, Ren L, Zhao J, Hu Y, Zhang L, Fan G, Xu J, Gu X, et al. Clinical features of patients infected with 2019 novel coronavirus in Wuhan, China. Lancet. 2020;395(10223):497–506.
63. Zumla A, Hui DS, Azhar EI, Memish ZA, Maeurer M. Reducing mortality from 2019-nCoV: host-directed therapies should be an option. Lancet. 2020;395(10224):e35–6.
64. Zeng F, Li L, Zeng J, et al. Can we predict the severity of coronavirus disease 2019 with a routine blood test?. Pol Arch Intern Med. 2020;130(5):400–6. https://doi.org/10.20452/pamw.15331.
65. Peng YD, Meng K, Guan HQ, Leng L, Zhu RR, Wang BY, He MA, Cheng LX, Huang K, Zeng QT. Clinical characteristics and outcomes of 112 cardiovascular disease patients infected by 2019-nCoV. Zhonghua Xin Xue Guan Bing Za Zhi. 2020;48:E004.
66. Qin C, Zhou L, Hu Z, et al. Dysregulation of Immune Response in Patients With Coronavirus 2019 (COVID-19) in Wuhan, China. Clin Infect Dis. 2020;71(15):762–8. https://doi.org/10.1093/cid/ciaa248.
67. Chen L, Liu HG, Liu W, Liu J, Liu K, Shang J, Deng Y, Wei S. Analysis of clinical features of 29 patients with 2019 novel coronavirus pneumonia. Zhonghua Jie He He Hu Xi Za Zhi. 2020;43(3):203–8.
68. Bai X, Fang C, Zhou Y, Bai S, Liu Z, Chen Q, Xu Y, Xia T, Gong S, Xie X et al. Predicting COVID-19 malignant progression with AI techniques. medRxiv 2020:2020.03.20.20037325.

69. Yan L, Zhang H-T, Goncalves J, Xiao Y, Wang M, Guo Y, Sun C, Tang X, Jin L, Zhang M et al. A machine learning-based model for survival prediction in patients with severe COVID-19 infection. medRxiv 2020:2020.02.27.20028027.

70. Wynants L, Van Calster B, Bonten MMJ, Collins GS, Debray TPA, De Vos M, Haller MC, Heinze G, Moons KGM, Riley RD, et al. Prediction models for diagnosis and prognosis of covid-19 infection: systematic review and critical appraisal. BMJ. 2020;369:m1328.

71. Ji D, Zhang D, Xu J, et al. Prediction for Progression Risk in Patients with COVID-19 Pneumonia: the CALL Score [published online ahead of print, 2020 Apr 9]. Clin Infect Dis. 2020;ciaa414. https://doi.org/10.1093/cid/ciaa414.

72. Liang W, Liang H, Ou L, et al. Development and Validation of a Clinical Risk Score to Predict the Occurrence of Critical Illness in Hospitalized Patients With COVID-19 [published online ahead of print, 2020 May 12]. J AMA Intern Med. 2020;e202033. https://doi.org/10.1001/jamainternmed.2020.2033.

73. Zou X, Li S, Fang M, et al. Acute Physiology and Chronic Health Evaluation II Score as a Predictor of Hospital Mortality in Patients of Coronavirus Disease 2019 [published online ahead of print, 2020 May 1]. Crit Care Med. 2020;48(8):e657–e665. https://doi.org/10.1097/CCM.0000000000004411.

74. Hui DS, Joynt GM, Wong KT, Gomersall CD, Li TS, Antonio G, Ko FW, Chan MC, Chan DP, Tong MW, et al. Impact of severe acute respiratory syndrome (SARS) on pulmonary function, functional capacity and quality of life in a cohort of survivors. Thorax. 2005;60(5):401–9.

Elderly Pneumonia COVID-19 Cases: Impact on the Outcome

2

Loredana Tibullo, Dalila Bruno, Emanuela Landi, Giovanni Carifi, Filomena Micillo, Elisa Salsano, and Maria Amitrano

2.1 Introduction

In elderly, pneumonia may be more severe because of impaired immunity and frailty as well as a reduced ability to cough and clear secretions from the lungs. Hence, they have an increased rate of respiratory failure and death. Furthermore, the impact of COVID-19 pneumonia in the elderly may have the characteristics of a multisystem disease with direct consequences on the treatment. Pneumonia in elderly patients with multimorbidity is significantly more complicated. For these reasons, the rate of hospitalisation and the mortality rate is very high in older patients. The presence of comorbidities, as well as a frailty condition, is a risk factor. The most common symptoms on admission were fever and cough, followed by sputum production and fatigue [1]. Elderly may present an atypical presentation of the

L. Tibullo (✉)
Medicine Department, Ward of Internal Medicine, San Giuseppe Moscati Hospital, Aversa, Italy

D. Bruno
Department of Translational Medical Sciences, Federico II University, Naples, Italy

E. Landi · G. Carifi
Department of Medicine, Geriatric and Intensive Geriatric Cares, San Giuseppe Moscati Hospital, Avellino, Italy

F. Micillo
Medicine Department, Maresca Hospital, Torre del Greco, Naples, Italy

E. Salsano
Geriatric Ward, Ospedale di Circolo, ASST Settelaghi, Varese, Italy

M. Amitrano
Medicine Department, Medicine Ward, San Giuseppe Moscati Hospital, Avellino, Italy

15

N. Vargas, A. M. Esquinas (eds.), *Covid-19 Airway Management and Ventilation Strategy for Critically Ill Older Patients*, https://doi.org/10.1007/978-3-030-55621-1_2

symptoms. But they are more susceptible to severe complications that may lead to death. In this chapter, the authors analysed the type and the impact of complications in elderly patients.

2.2　Acute Complications Associated with COVID-19 Pneumonia in Elderly

Generally, the majority of studies reported that patients with severe disease were older than those with nonsevere [2]. In 15–30% of case series of patients with pneumonia COVID-19, the most acute complication has been the acute respiratory distress syndrome (ARDS), which is a type of respiratory failure characterised by rapid onset of widespread inflammation in the lungs and also defined [3–5]. A case report of an oldest-old patient with pneumonia COVID-19 developed ARDS in the course of a few days. The patient presented the development of bilateral lung opacities and arterial blood gas analysis rapidly yielding a reduced pO_2/FiO_2 ratio. Respiratory failure dominated the clinical picture throughout his illness, with only a minor degree of other organ affection. After broad multidisciplinary discussion, and in consultation with his family, the physicians decided that, given the patient's advanced age, pronounced comorbidity and very rapid disease progression, ventilator treatment should not be offered [6]. Furthermore, according to a report of Italian Istituto Superiore di Sanità the most acute conditions observed in elderly patients with COVID-19 pneumonia were: acute respiratory distress syndrome (ARDS) found in the majority of patients (96.5% of cases); acute renal failure (29.2%); severe cardiac injury observed in 10.4% of cases and superinfection in 8.5% [7]. Many elderly patients who had severe hypoxaemia also presented with hypotension. These patients required intubation, and 2% had cardiac arrest and pneumothorax [8]. Liu et al. [9] showed that in the elderly group, pneumonia had more multiple lobe involvement than that in the young and middle-aged group. The ARDS, acute heart, liver and kidney failure in the elderly group were higher than that in the young and middle-aged group. The authors found that elderly patients are inclined to multisystem organ failure. The authors found that elderly patients are inclined to multisystem organ dysfunction and even failure. Systemic complications should be prevented, including gastrointestinal bleeding, renal failure, disseminated intravascular coagulation (DIC) or deep vein thrombosis, delirium and secondary infections.

2.3　Elderly Mortality Rate for COVID-19 Disease

Data from COVID-NET suggest that COVID-19-associated hospitalisations in the United States are highest among older adults, and nearly 90% of persons hospitalised have one or more underlying medical conditions (Fig. 2.1) [10]. The Italian Istituto Superiore di Sanità in a recent report stated that the mean age of patients

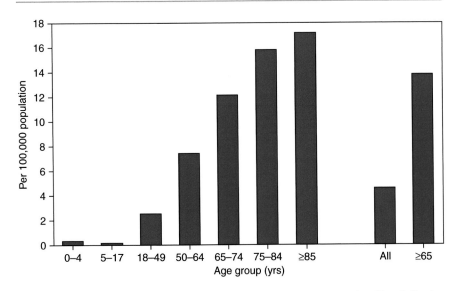

Fig. 2.1 Laboratory-confirmed coronavirus disease 2019 (COVID-19)-associated hospitalization rates, "by age group—COVID-NET, 14 states,† March 1–28, 2020. Abbreviation: *COVID-NET* Coronovirus Disease 2019–Associated Hospitalization Surveillance Network.

dying of COVID-2019 infection was 78.5. Also, the studies established that men die more than women in the elder age group [7]. In a retrospective case study with 52 critically ill patients, elderly patients had higher mortality associated with comorbidity and ARDS. After 28 days, 61.5% of the patients in the study had died. The elderly patients who died developed ARDS (81%) more frequently than those who survived (45%). Of these patients, only two in the study were ≥80 years old, and both died [11]. THE WHO data demonstrated that over 95% of deaths occurred in those older than 60 years. More than 50% of all fatalities involved people aged 80 years or older. Reports show that 8 out of 10 deaths are occurring in individuals with at least one comorbidity, in particular, those with cardiovascular disease, hypertension and diabetes, but also with a range of other chronic underlying conditions [12].

2.4   Conclusion

The impact of COVID-19 pneumonia on the elderly is severe. The fatal cases are high. The negative outcome is mainly due to the incidence of complications and between these to the ARDS. The action of the COVID pneumonia is primary a multisystemic disease with involving many organs. The multiorgan failure in elderly patients has a high mortality rate. The preventive measure should be robust in this group of patients as well as the possibility of adequate intensive caring through a multidisciplinary team.

References

1. Zhou F, Yu T, Du R, et al. Clinical course and risk factors for mortality of adult inpatients with COVID-19 in Wuhan, China: a retrospective cohort study. Lancet. 2020;395:P1054–62.
2. Guan W-j, Ni Z-y, Hu Y, Liang W-h, Ou C-q, He J-x, Liu L, Shan H, Lei C-l, Hui DSC, Du B, Li L-j, Zeng et al. for the China Medical Treatment Expert Group for Covid-19. Clinical Characteristics of Coronavirus Disease 2019 in China. N Engl J Med. 2020;382:1708–20. https://doi.org/10.1056/NEJMoa2002032.
3. Huang C, Wang Y, Li X, et al. Clinical features of patients infected with 2019 novel coronavirus in Wuhan, China. Lancet. 2020;395:497–506.
4. Chen N, Zhou M, Dong X, et al. Epidemiological and clinical characteristics of 99 cases of 2019 novel coronavirus pneumonia in Wuhan, China: a descriptive study. Lancet. 2020;395:507–13.
5. Wang D, Hu B, Hu C, et al. Clinical characteristics of 138 hospitalized patients with 2019 novel coronavirus-infected pneumonia in Wuhan, China. JAMA. 2020;323:1061–9.
6. Borén HK, Kjøstolfsen GH, Aaløkken TM, Latif N, Brekke H, Lind A, Hesstvedt L. A man in his nineties with fever and dry cough. Tidsskr Nor Laegeforen. 2020;140:6. https://doi.org/10.4045/tidsskr.20.0218.
7. Available at https://www.epicentro.iss.it/coronavirus/bollettino/Report-COVID-2019_20_marzo_eng.pdf.
8. Yao W, Peng Z, et al. Emergency tracheal intubation in 202 patients with COVID-19 in Wuhan, China: lessons learnt and international expert recommendations. Br J Anaesth. 2020;125(1):E28–37.
9. Liu K, Chen Y, Lin R, Han K. Clinical features of COVID-19 in elderly patients: a comparison with young and middle-aged patients. J Inf Secur. 2020;80(6):e14–8. https://doi.org/10.1016/j.jinf.2020.03.005.
10. Garg S, Kim L, Whitaker M, et al. Hospitalization rates and characteristics of patients hospitalized with laboratory-confirmed coronavirus disease 2019—COVID-NET, 14 States, March 1–30, 2020. Morb Mortal Wkly Rep. 2020;69:458–64. https://doi.org/10.15585/mmwr.mm6915e3.
11. Yang X, Yu Y, Xu J, et al. Clinical course and outcomes of critically ill patients with SARS-CoV2 pneumonia in Wuhan, China: a single-centered, retrospective, observational study. Lancet. 2020;395:475. https://doi.org/10.1016/S2213-2600(20)30079-5.
12. http://www.euro.who.int/en/health-topics/health-emergencies/coronavirus-covid19/news/news/2020/4/supporting-older-people-during-the-covid-19-pandemic-is-everyones-business.

Incidence of ARF Due to COVID-19 Interstitial Pneumonia

Annamaria Romano and Antonio Vitale

Since November 2019 and starting from the Chinese region of Wuhan, the severe acute respiratory syndrome-coronavirus-2 (SARS-CoV-2), a novel coronavirus capable of infecting humans, has developed and spread worldwide showing to induce an unprecedented clinical condition defined COronaVIrus Disease 2019 (COVID-19).

SARS-CoV-2 infection may lead to a protean spectrum of clinical manifestations that may bring about five different outcomes: asymptomatical condition (1.2–17.9%), that is as high as 15.8% among children aged under 10 years old [1]; mild to medium disease (about 80%); severe cases (about 14%); critical cases (4.7–6.1%), and death (1.4–4.5% according to different cohorts) [2, 3]. Therefore, COVID-19 may induce a serious or critical clinical picture in a not negligible percentage of patients resulting in a significant mortality rate and an overloading of national health systems.

Clinical manifestations of SARS-CoV-2 infection appear after an incubation period of approximately 5.2 days [4]. Symptoms more frequently encountered in COVID-19 patients are fever (88.7–98.8%), cough (57.6–76%), and myalgia or fatigue (29.4–42.5%), while sputum production (28%), headache (8%), hemoptysis (5%), and diarrhea (3%) are less frequent. Respiratory symptoms are prominent manifestations in hospitalized COVID-19 patients: in addition to cough and sputum production, dyspnea is observed in up to half of patients [5–8], while acute respiratory distress syndrome (ARDS) is the most frequent complication among patients experiencing a negative outcome [9].

A. Romano (✉)
Division of Respiratory Medicine, San Giuseppe Moscati Hospital, Avellino, Italy

A. Vitale
Research Center of Systemic Autoinflammatory Diseases and Behçet's Disease Clinic, Department of Medical Sciences, Surgery and Neurosciences, University of Siena, Siena, Italy

ARDS is a well-known life-threatening condition preventing enough oxygen from getting to the lungs and into the circulation. It is closely related to genetic susceptibility and pro-inflammatory cytokines, as more than 40 candidate genes, including ACE2, interleukin-10, and tumor necrosis factor, have been associated with the development or outcome of ARDS [10]. ARDS and hypoxemic respiratory failure may be found in 60–89.9% of patients who die during hospitalization, thus representing the leading cause of death and a top priority complication in case of SARS-CoV-2 infection [9, 11, 12].

To date, there is a wide range in the reported incidence of ARDS among patients with COVID-19: while initial studies from Wuhan in China reported an incidence ranging from 17% to 29% [7, 13–15], the reported incidence of ARDS in areas away from the epicenter of the first disease outbreak appears to be significantly lower, falling below 3% [16–18]. Nevertheless, in all these studies the incidence of ARDS may be underestimated, as the majority of patients remained hospitalized at the time of analysis. Moreover, different hospitalization policies may have significantly affected results about ARDS incidences. In order to reduce these biases, data from meta-analysis may be considered: according to Sun et al., when based on 10 studies (9 from China and 1 from America) enrolling 50,466 patients, the incidence of ARDS was 14.8%, while the fatality rate was 4.3% in the whole cohort [5]. A second meta-analysis proposed by Zhu et al. and based on 38 cohort studies, case-control studies, and case series studies (all conducted in China) found that the incidence of respiratory failure or ARDS was 19.5% in 3062 hospitalized COVID-19 patients, while the fatality rate was 5.5% [19]. A further meta-analysis by Rodriguez-Morales et al. identified ARDS in 32.8% of patients requiring intensive care with a fatality rate of 13.9% among hospitalized patients. In this case, a third of patients with complications and death presented with ARDS [6].

As much for the time of ARDS presentation, it tends to occur about 8–14 days after the onset of COVID-19 symptoms and is often precipitous and protracted and may require high-flow nasal cannula, non-invasive mechanical ventilation up to early intubation. In this regard, intubation has been required in 10–33% of cases according to various Chinese series [20, 21].

When trying to early identify patients more likely developing ARDS, older age (especially ≥65 years), preexisting concurrent cardiovascular or cerebrovascular diseases, baseline hypertension, diabetes, high fever, injury to other organs (such as acute kidney disease), lymphopenia, decreased fibrinogen levels, and elevated d-dimer, C-reactive protein, ferritin serum levels, transaminases, and lactate dehydrogenase represent predictors of ARDS. Of note, older age, neutropenia, CD3[+] CD8[+] T cells ≤75, increased d-dimer, cardiac troponin I (≥0.05 ng/mL), and inflammatory markers are associated with higher mortality in patients with ARDS [20, 22]. Interestingly, patients who produce neutralizing antibodies early seem to be more susceptible to the development of acute respiratory symptoms. This phenomenon, also described for other coronavirus infections, is an antibody-dependent enhancement of inflammation induced by the uptake of virus–antibody complexes in target immune cells [23].

Noteworthy, development of ARDS itself represents an independent predictor of death along with the occurrence of acute cardiac injury. The mean time from the onset of COVID-19 symptoms to death ranged from 6 to 41 days with a median of 14–18 days. This period is shorter among patients older than 70 years [3, 14]. The estimated case fatality ratio is lower among patients aged under 60 years (about 1.4%) when compared to subjects aged 60 years and over (4.5–6.4%); specifically, the estimated case fatality ratio results lowest in the 0–9 years age group (very close to 0%) and highest in the 80 years and older age group (13.4%). In parallel, the percentage of infected individuals requiring hospitalization was the lowest in the 0–9 years age group (0.00%) and highest among patients aged ≥80 years (18.4%) [3].

Based on these data, the overall mortality rate of SARS-CoV-2 is lower than that reported for other coronaviruses determining lung involvement (10% mortality for SARS-CoV, that is the causative agent of a viral outbreak in 2002, and 37.1% for the Middle East respiratory syndrome coronavirus); nonetheless, the number of relative SARS-COV-2 infection cases is more than 10 times higher, likewise making this pandemic a major public health issue.

With regard to the frequency of typical COVID-19 findings at chest computed tomography (CT) images, early stage findings include ground-glass opacities with rare small-size consolidations mainly distributed in the peripheral and posterior part of the lungs, while bilateral involvement is found in up to 98% of patients under chest CT [24]. On hospital admission, CT findings are mainly represented by bilateral multiple lobular and subsegmental areas of consolidation for patients needing intensive care; bilateral ground-glass opacity and subsegmental areas of consolidation are more typical findings in patients not requiring admission to intensive care units [7].

In conclusion, COVID-19 is a protean condition that may lead to severe or critical disease in a not negligible percentage of patients. In this context, ARDS accounts for a primary cause of admission to intensive care units and represents the leading cause of death among subjects with SARS-CoV-2 infection, especially in elderly people and in case of underlying comorbidities. Future studies are required to clearly define clinical, laboratory, and radiological features capable to early recognize patients at high risk to develop serious complications. Moreover, future research efforts should aim at understanding why some COVID-19 patients experience persistent inflammation, ARDS, and even death, while most of patients survive the inflammatory response and clear the virus more easily.

References

1. Lu X, Zhang L, Du H, Zhang J, Li YY, Qu J, et al. SARS-CoV-2 infection in children. N Engl J Med. 2020;382:1663–5. https://doi.org/10.1056/NEJMc2005073.
2. Mizumoto K, Kagaya K, Zarebski A, Chowell G. Estimating the asymptomatic proportion of coronavirus disease 2019 (COVID-19) cases on board the diamond princess cruise ship, Yokohama, Japan, 2020. Euro Surveill. 2020;25:2000180. https://doi.org/10.2807/1560-7917. ES.2020.25.10.2000180.

3. Verity R, Okell LC, Dorigatti I, Winskill P, Whittaker C, Imai N, et al. Estimates of the severity of coronavirus disease 2019: a model-based analysis. Lancet Infect Dis. 2020;20:669. https://doi.org/10.1016/S1473-3099(20)30243-7.
4. Li Q, Guan X, Wu P, Wang X, Zhou L, Tong Y, et al. Early transmission dynamics in Wuhan, China, of novel coronavirus-infected pneumonia. N Engl J Med. 2020;382:1199–207.
5. Sun P, Qie S, Liu Z, Ren J, Li K, Xi J. Clinical characteristics of hospitalized patients with SARS-CoV-2 infection: a single arm meta-analysis. J Med Virol. 2020;92:612. https://doi.org/10.1002/jmv.25735.
6. Rodriguez-Morales AJ, Cardona-Ospina JA, Gutiérrez-Ocampo E, Villamizar-Peña R, Holguin-Rivera Y, Escalera-Antezana JP, et al. Clinical, laboratory and imaging features of COVID-19: a systematic review and meta-analysis. Travel Med Infect Dis. 2020;24:101623. https://doi.org/10.1016/j.tmaid.2020.101623.
7. Huang C, Wang Y, Li X, Ren L, Zhao J, Hu Y, et al. Clinical features of patients infected with 2019 novel coronavirus in Wuhan, China. Lancet. 2020;395:497–506. https://doi.org/10.1016/S0140-6736(20)30183-5.
8. Wang W, Tang J, Wei F. Updated understanding of the outbreak of 2019 novel coronavirus (2019-nCoV) in Wuhan, China. J Med Virol. 2020;92:441–7. https://doi.org/10.1002/jmv.25689.
9. Deng Y, Liu W, Liu K, Fang YY, Shang J, Zhou L, et al. Clinical characteristics of fatal and recovered cases of coronavirus disease 2019 (COVID-19) in Wuhan, China: a retrospective study. Chin Med J. 2020;133:1261. https://doi.org/10.1097/CM9.0000000000000824.
10. Meyer NJ, Christie JD. Genetic heterogeneity and risk of acute respiratory distress syndrome. Semin Respir Crit Care Med. 2013;34:459–74. https://doi.org/10.1055/s-0033-1351121.
11. Shi S, Qin M, Shen B, Cai Y, Liu T, Yang F, et al. Association of Cardiac Injury with Mortality in hospitalized patients with COVID-19 in Wuhan, China. JAMA Cardiol. 2020;2020:e200950. https://doi.org/10.1001/jamacardio.2020.0950.
12. Ruan Q, Yang K, Wang W, Jiang L, Song J. Clinical predictors of mortality due to COVID-19 based on an analysis of data of 150 patients from Wuhan, China. Intens Care Med. 2020;46:846. https://doi.org/10.1007/s00134-020-05991-x.
13. Chen N, Zhou M, Dong X, Qu J, Gong F, Han Y, et al. Epidemiological and clinical characteristics of 99 cases of 2019 novel coronavirus pneumonia in Wuhan, China: a descriptive study. Lancet. 2020;395:507–13. https://doi.org/10.1016/S0140-6736(20)30211-7.
14. Wang D, Hu B, Hu C, Zhu F, Liu X, Zhang J, et al. Clinical characteristics of 138 hospitalized patients with 2019 novel coronavirus-infected pneumonia in Wuhan, China. JAMA. 2020;323:1061. https://doi.org/10.1001/jama.2020.1585.
15. Yang X, Yu Y, Xu J, Shu H, Xia J, Liu H, et al. Clinical course and outcomes of critically ill patients with SARS-CoV-2 pneumonia in Wuhan, China: a single-centered, retrospective, observational study. Lancet Respir Med. 2020;8:475. https://doi.org/10.1016/S2213-2600(20)30079-5.
16. Guan WJ, Ni ZY, Hu Y, Liang WH, Ou CQ, He JX, et al. Clinical characteristics of coronavirus disease 2019 in China. N Engl J Med. 2020;382:1708. https://doi.org/10.1056/NEJMoa2002032.
17. Xu XW, Wu XX, Jiang XG, Xu KJ, Ying LJ, Ma CL, et al. Clinical findings in a group of patients infected with the 2019 novel coronavirus (SARS-Cov-2) outside of Wuhan, China: retrospective case series. BMJ. 2020;368:m606. https://doi.org/10.1136/bmj.m606.
18. Wu J, Liu J, Zhao X, Liu C, Wang W, Wang D, et al. Clinical characteristics of imported cases of COVID-19 in Jiangsu Province: a multicenter descriptive study. Clin Infect Dis. 2020;2020:ciaa199. https://doi.org/10.1093/cid/ciaa199.
19. Zhu J, Ji P, Pang J, Zhong Z, Li H, He C, et al. Clinical characteristics of 3,062 COVID-19 patients: a meta-analysis. J Med Virol. 2020; https://doi.org/10.1002/jmv.25884.
20. Wu C, Chen X, Cai Y, Xia J, Zhou X, Xu S, et al. Risk factors associated with acute respiratory distress syndrome and death in patients with coronavirus disease 2019 pneumonia in Wuhan, China. JAMA Intern Med. 2020; https://doi.org/10.1001/jamainternmed.2020.0994.

21. Zhou F, Yu T, Du R, Fan G, Liu Y, Liu Z, et al. Clinical course and risk factors for mortality of adult inpatients with COVID-19 in Wuhan, China: a retrospective cohort study. Lancet. 2020;395:1054–62. https://doi.org/10.1016/S0140-6736(20)30566-3.
22. Du RH, Liang LR, Yang CQ, Wang W, Cao TZ, Li M, et al. Predictors of mortality for patients with COVID-19 pneumonia caused by SARS-CoV-2: a prospective cohort study. Eur Respir J. 2020;55:2000524. https://doi.org/10.1183/13993003.00524-2020.
23. Fu Y, Cheng Y, Wu Y. Understanding SARS-CoV-2-mediated inflammatory responses: from mechanisms to potential therapeutic tools. Virol Sin. 2020; https://doi.org/10.1007/s12250-020-00207-4.
24. Yang S, Shi Y, Lu H, Xu J, Li F, Qian Z, et al. Clinical and CT features of early-stage patients with COVID-19: a retrospective analysis of imported cases in Shanghai, China. Eur Respir J. 2020;55:2000407. https://doi.org/10.1183/13993003.00407-2020.

Changing the Demographics in ICU During COVID-19 Pandemic

4

Maria Vargas, Rosario Sara, Carmine Iacovazzo, and Giuseppe Servillo

The improvement in clinical care pathways, socioeconomic conditions, and behavioral habits has been responsible for the incredible increase in life expectancy between the two centuries.

This, by increasing the number of the population in the elderly age group, has both exposed to acute conditions a population with increasingly worn homeostatic mechanisms and reduced the stringent inclusion criteria in intensive unit care. In this sense, Europe represents the continent with the highest aging index [1].

According to Eurostat data, updated to 1 January 2018, in the 27 countries of the European Union 19.7% of the total population is over 65 years of age (with an increase of 0.3% points compared to the previous year and 2, 6 compared to 10 years earlier).

In the period between 2018 and 2100, the share of the working-age population is expected to continue to decrease until 2100, while the elderly will probably represent an increasing share of the total population (Fig. 4.1): people aged 65 and over will constitute 31.3% of the EU-28 population in 2100. As regards access to the emergency department, a share of more than 15% is made up of a population of over 65 who tend to be even the most complex users. Of 40% of patients admitted to hospital, 15% were admitted to ICU. Beyond the possibility that some elderly people resort to the emergency department for lack of responses at the level of primary care, the need for ICU admission is often real [2].

The need to renew and strengthen the ICUs and SICUs is evident on the basis of these data and the problems born with the COVID-19 epidemic.

M. Vargas (✉) · R. Sara · C. Iacovazzo · G. Servillo
Department of Neurosciences, Reproductive Sciences and Odontostomatology,
University of Naples Federico II, Naples, Italy

N. Vargas, A. M. Esquinas (eds.), *Covid-19 Airway Management and Ventilation Strategy for Critically Ill Older Patients*, https://doi.org/10.1007/978-3-030-55621-1_4

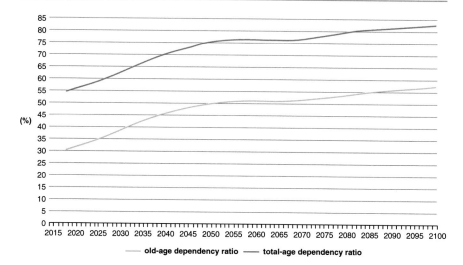

Fig. 4.1 Projected total-age and old-age dependency ratio, EU–28, 2018–2100; Eurostat

4.1   Pre-COVID-19 Epidemy Demographic Aspects in ICU

The increase in life expectancy observed in the world over recent years means that the average age of patients being admitted to an intensive care unit (ICU) has increased considerably.

In recent decades, the rate curve of the population aged over 75 has clearly came near the rate curve of elderly patients hospitalized in the ICU (Fig. 4.2).

Elderly patients above the age of 75 years already represent the largest group of patients admitted to the ICU setting [4].

As a consequence of people getting older and older, it can be expected that much more patients will need intensive care support during their hospital stay [5].

Jones et al. in a demographic analysis involving many European and non-European countries have shown that the UK data are superimposable on the rest of the countries.

Excluding readmissions within the same hospital stay, there were 318,621 patients admitted to general ICUs in England, Wales, and Northern Ireland. Of these, 24.4% patients were 65–74 years, 19.9% were 75–84 years, and 5.8% were 85 years old or older.

The proportion of older patients admitted following emergency surgery was highest in the age bands of 75–84 years and 85 years old or older [3].

However, while more and more people survive to acute critical situations, the developments in the organ support can lead to a state called "chronic critical illness" [6].

An unreflected application of intensive care measures might lead to prolonged treatment for incurable diseases, and an inadequate or too aggressive

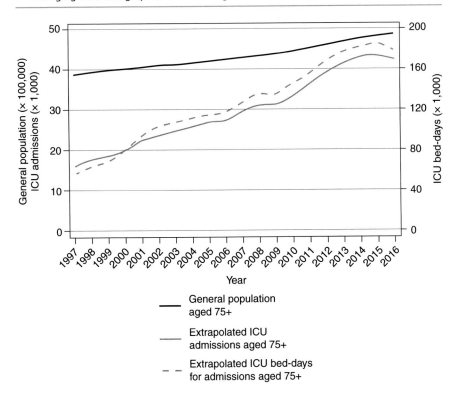

Fig. 4.2 The extrapolated rate of ICU admissions for patients 75 years old or older relative to the general population [3]

therapy can prolong the dying process. Due to the increasing number of patients dying in ICUs, there has been a lot of discussion about end-of-life decisions in intensive care units and how much and what intensity of care is in patient's best interest [7].

Regarding gender distribution, approximately 52% of the patients who had access to intensive care were male. More precisely, between the ages of 65 and 74 years (young older), 57.9% of males were hospitalized, in the age group between 75 and 84 years 56.0%, and the old older males amounted to 49.1%.

The comorbidities were the main determinants of mortality and duration of hospitalization. The geriatric patients admitted to ICU were mainly (only conclaime diseases): very severe cardio' comorbidities were: - vascular disease (2.8%; 2.2% in youngest old people, 2.9% in middle old, 3.3% in oldest old); - severe respiratory disease (2.7%; 3.4%, 2.7%, 1.6%); - chronic renal replacement therapy (2.1%; 2.3%, 1.9%, 1.1%), and liver disease (0.9%; 1.7, 0.9%, 0.3%) [3, 8].

Geriatric patients were admitted to ICU for clinical problems in 49.4% of cases (52.7%, 51.4, 49.7%), following elective surgery in 26.6% of cases (30.1%, 27.3%, 22.5%) and for emergency surgery in 23.2% of cases (17.3%, 21.6%, and 30.1%) [9].

4.2 Demographic Aspects During the COVID-19 Outbreak in ICU

The novel coronavirus 2019 is a disease that has affected populations around the world because it is caused by a highly contagious virus that has spread rapidly and efficiently.

As of April 16, 2020, there are 1,991,562 confirmed cases and 130,885 deaths from Sars-Cov2. In the 27 EU member states there are 1,013,093 cases and 89,371 deaths while in Italy alone 165,155 cases with 21,647 deaths [10].

The data on the gender difference of the infected in the world show a fair preference for the male gender 59.8% vs. 40.2% for female gender.

The evident high lethality rate of this pathology, in addition to having to manage a disease with unusual clinical-pathological characteristics, could not fail to have implications for the organization and management of ICUs all over the world. During the COVID-19 epidemic, the proportion of ICU admissions represents in Italy the 12% of the total positive cases, and 16% of all hospitalized patients. This rate is higher than what was reported from China, where only 5% of patients who tested positive for COVID-19 required ICU admission.

In the USA, 35% of COVID-19 patients had access to intensive care [11].

There could be different explanations. It is possible that criteria for ICU admission were different between the countries, but this seems unlikely. Another explanation is that the Italian and American population is different from the Chinese population, with predisposing factors such as race, age, and comorbidities [12].

The median age of hospitalization in the ICU was found to be overlapping in all three main countries involved: the most affected population group is between 56 and 70 years of age.

In the USA, COVID-19 hospitalized patients with access in ICU aged ≥85 years were 7%; 46% among adults aged 65–84 years, 36% among adults aged 45–64 years, and 11% among adults aged 20–44 years [11]. In Italy, these proportions are slightly different: 2% of the patients hospitalized for COVID-19 who entered the ICU were over the age of 80 (aged > 84 years); 21% were in the 75–84 age group. As many as 38% of intensive care was reserved for COVID-19 patients between 60 and 74 years while 27% of these patients were in the age group between 51 and 60 years. The remaining 12% of ICU logins were accounted for patients under 50 years of age [12].

As for the breakdown by age of accesses in ICU, the Chinese data overlap the trends of western countries [13]. As regards the gender distribution, the differences with the pre-epidemic prospectus are even more clear.

Therefore during the COVID-19 epidemic, the youngest old patients had less access to intensive care for a greater attention for middle old and patients aged <65 years (Fig. 4.3). This data reflects the average age of the disease and certain

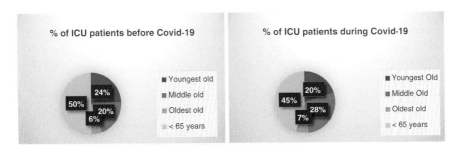

Fig. 4.3 Comparison between epidemiological data in ICU before and during COVID-19 in Anglo-Saxon countries

choices based on ensuring the best expectation and quality of life in this emergency period.

An average (among the data of the main countries involved) of 82% of patients hospitalized and then hospitalized in ICU is male with a homogeneous distribution in the various age groups (83% of males between 51 and 70 years of age, 82% between 71 and 80 years, and 92% over 80) [11, 12].

COVID-positive patients who access intensive care in 78% of cases experience more than one comorbidity. Hypertension and hypercholesterolemia are more frequent with a prevalence, respectively, of 49% and 18%. Cardiovascular disease (including cardiomyopathy and heart failure) are present in 40% of patients while 17% of patients have diabetes type 2.

The youngest old COVID positives accepted in ICU have hypertension, 23% hypercholesterolemia, 24% cardiovascular disease, and diabetes in 23% of cases. As regards the gender distribution, the differences with the pre-epidemic prospectus are even more clear [11, 12].

On the other hand, the middle old patients have hypertension and cardiovascular disease, respectively, in 64% and 32% of cases. Hypercholesterolemia is present in 23% of these patients and diabetes types 2 in 18% of the same. The elderly have hypertension in 75% of cases and cardiovascular disease in 38% of cases. Hypercholesterolemia is present in 31% of these patients and diabetes types 2 in 19% of the same.

4.3 Comparison between H1N1 and COVID-19 Epidemy

Between 2009 and 2010, the national health system had to face a flu pandemic caused by Orthomyxoviridae H1N1.

The clinical and therapeutic aspects of this pandemic have numerous common factors with the Sars-CoV-2: respiratory tropism, hyperactivation of the inflammatory chain, tendency to ARDS, and need for ventilatory support and/or ECMO.

Furthermore, both started in the East world.

The median age of patients with COVID-19 was 67 years, which was significantly higher than that of patients with H1N1 (52 years). The proportion of male subjects in the COVID-19 group was 61.5%, which was significantly lower than that of the H1N1 group (80.0%) [14].

In terms of underlying diseases, 31.5% of COVID-19 patients has a history of cardiovascular disease, whereas that of H1N1 patients was significantly lower (10.7%). There was no significant difference in the history of hypertension, diabetes, or chronic airway diseases.

During the H1N1 global epidemic in 2009, Jain et al. found that 5% of patients with H1N1 influenza were admitted to ICUs [15].

These data compared with the heterogeneous data from the main countries affected by COVID-19 (from 5% of access to China's ICU up to more than 30% of accesses in the USA) give an idea of how much the latter agent has a contagiousness and a pathogenicity such as to require a strengthening of the ICU offer.

4.4 Conclusions

The increase in life expectancy observed in the world over recent years means that the average age of patients being admitted to an intensive care unit has increased considerably.

During COVID-19 pandemic the median age of hospitalization in the ICU was found to be overlapping in all three main countries involved since the most affected population group is between 56 and 70 years of age.

References

1. Antonelli I, Cesari R, et al. Societa' Ital; Manuale di geriatria. 2019, Edra–Masson.
2. Zincarelli C, Ferrara N, Rengo G. Intensive care for the elderly: between outcome and ethics. G Gerontol. 2011;59:191–7.
3. Andrew Jones MD, Toft-Petersen AP, Shankar-Hari M, Harrison DA, Rowan KM. Demographic shifts, case mix, activity, and outcome for elderly patients admitted to adult general ICUs in England, Wales, and Northern Ireland. Crit Care Med. 2020;48:4.
4. McDermid RC, Bagshaw SM. ICU and critical care outreach for the elderly. Best Pract Res Clin Anaesthesiol. 2011;25:439–49.
5. Ay E, Weigand MA, Röhrig R, Gruss M. Dying in the Intensive Care Unit (ICU): a retrospective descriptive analysis of deaths in the ICU in a communal tertiary Hospital in Germany. Anesthesiol Res Pract. 2020;2020:2356019.
6. Lamas DJ, Owens RL, Nace RN, et al. Opening the door. Crit Care Med. 2017;45(4):e357–62.
7. Hillman K, Athari F, Forero R. States worse than death. Curr Opin Crit Care. 2018;24(5):415–20.
8. Vargas N. Et al; caring for critically ill oldest old patients: a clinical review. Aging Clin Exp Res. 2017 Oct;29(5):833–45.
9. Agodi A, et al. Epidemiology of intensive care unit-acquired sepsis in Italy: results of the SPIN-UTI network. Ann Ig. 2018;30:15–21.
10. Coronavirus Disease 2019 (COVID-19) Situation Report—87. World Health Organization.

11. US Department of Health and Human Services Severe Outcomes among Patients with Coronavirus Disease 2019 (COVID-19)—March 27, 2020/Vol. 69/No. 12.
12. Grasselli G et al. Critical Care Utilization for the COVID-19 Outbreak in Lombardy, Italy Early Experience and Forecast During an Emergency Response-JAMA Published online March 13, 2020.
13. Yang X, Yu Y, et al. Clinical course and outcomes of critically ill patients with SARS-CoV-2 pneumonia in Wuhan, China: a single-centered, retrospective, observational study. Lancet Respir Med. 2020;8(4):e26.
14. Tang X, Du R. Comparison of hospitalized patients with ARDS caused by COVID-19 and H1N1. Chest. 2020;158:195–205.
15. Jain S, Kamimoto L, Bramley AM, et al. Hospitalized patients with 2009 H1N1 influenza in the United States, April-June 2009. N Engl J Med. 2009;361(20):1935–44.

Part II

The Diagnosis of COVID ARF in Elderly

Differential Diagnosis of Types of Pneumonia in the Elderly

5

Attilio De Blasio, Laura Chioni, and Giuditta Adorni

5.1 Introduction

The lungs continue to develop throughout life reaching their maximal functional status in the early third decade and thereafter a gradual decline. Normal physiological and structural changes occur in the respiratory system with aging. Anatomical changes in both lungs and chest wall with multiple changes in structure and function give rise to changes in pulmonary mechanics, respiratory muscle strength and ventilation control. In spite of these changes, the gas exchange is adequately maintained. Age-related changes in pulmonary function result in decrease in respiratory reserve during acute illness. Changes occur in the pulmonary vasculature resulting in increase in pulmonary vascular stiffness, vascular pressures and vascular resistance. [1, 2].

- Anatomical changes result in changes in pulmonary mechanics, respiratory muscle strength and ventilation control.
- Changes in pulmonary function result in decrease in respiratory reserve during acute illness.
- Changes in pulmonary vasculature result in increase in pulmonary vascular stiffness, vascular pressures and vascular resistance.
- Thickening of the alveolar basement membrane results in decrease gas diffusing capabilities and increase in ventilation/perfusion heterogeneity.
- Decrease in small airway diameter gives an obstructive flow pattern.
- The conduction zone increases in size resulting in increased residual volume and functional residual capacity and decreased vital capacity.

A. De Blasio (✉) · L. Chioni · G. Adorni
Emergency Department, Emergency Medicine and Emergency Room, Azienda Ospedaliero Univeritaria Hospital, Parma, Italy

© The Editor(s) (if applicable) and The Author(s), under exclusive license to
Springer Nature Switzerland AG 2020
N. Vargas, A. M. Esquinas (eds.), *Covid-19 Airway Management and Ventilation Strategy for Critically Ill Older Patients*, https://doi.org/10.1007/978-3-030-55621-1_5

35

Pneumonia is an infection or inflammation of one or both lungs. Pneumonia is one of the most common infections in the elderly. Approximately 20% of nosocomial infections in the elderly are due to pneumonia which is only second in prevalence to urinary tract infections [3, 4].

5.2 Aging of the Respiratory System and the Impact of Pneumonia

In the elderly there is a greater susceptibility to infection because of the age-related decline in immune response. Invasion by bacteria, viruses and other pathogens evokes a systemic inflammation in response to the active immune system. Innate immunity mechanisms include physical barriers and phagocytic cells such as neutrophils and macrophages which destroy the pathogenic bacteria. Elimination of bacteria is by activation of the phagocytes locally in the lung brought about by the innate defense mechanism. Structural changes occur with aging, for instance, there is a decrease in the cilia beat and numbers which reduces the clearance of debris and pathogens resulting in increased chance of infection. In the aged there is also a reduction in the total number of phagocytes resulting in their reduced bactericidal activity. During infection, antigen contact induces neutrophil activation and release of matrix metalloproteinases (MMPs) and possibly by setting off proinflammatory cytokines cause bacterial clearance. There is evidence that various levels of different MMPs have been detected in community-acquired and hospital-acquired pneumonias. Pulmonary inflammation may also be brought about by mechanical ventilation. Neutrophil recruitment with MMP release and activation induced by cytokine release may result in lung injury in this setting [5].

Pneumonia is an acute inflammation of the lungs caused by an infection. Usually, the initial diagnosis is based on chest X-ray and clinical findings. Causes, symptoms, treatment, preventive measures and prognosis differ if the infection is bacterial, mycobacterial, viral, fungal or parasitic; if it is acquired in an out-of-hospital setting, hospital or other treatment center; and if it develops in an immunocompetent or immunosuppressed patient.

Pneumonias have commonly been classified as hospital acquired or community acquired. Hospital-acquired pneumonia either appears 48 h or more after admission in a patient who did not already have or was not incubating pneumonia at the time of admission or develops soon after discharge from a hospital. All other pneumonias are considered to be community acquired.

Older adults make up the majority of patients actively treated in the healthcare system, in large part owing to their increased burden of chronic diseases but also because of their marked vulnerability to adverse health outcomes, such as functional and cognitive decline, falls, delirium, and frailty. This age-related vulnerability is thought to have its basis in altered biology that results in tissue and physiologic system changes, which in turn may contribute to many of these conditions and to the chronic disease states commonly seen in older adults. Importantly, these biologic changes are likely to be heterogeneous and to occur at different chronologic ages and in different organs at different rates. These complex age-related biologic changes represent a source of vulnerability that sets the stage for the marked increase in clinical sequelae observed in older adults.

The chest wall stiffens with advancing age, and the lungs lose elastic recoil. Maximal vital capacity declines by about 40%, but oxygen exchange declines by about 50% because of the additive effect of progressive ventilation-perfusion mismatching. As a result, the arterial PO_2 of many 80-year-olds is about 70–75 mmHg. The clinical manifestations are often progressive shortness of breath with exercise and an increased susceptibility to community-acquired pneumonia and even to aspiration pneumonia [4, 6].

5.3 Epidemiology

An estimated 2–3 million people in the USA contract pneumonia each year and 60,000 die of pneumonia. In the USA, pneumonia, along with flu, is the eighth leading cause of death and is the leading cause of death from infection. Pneumonia is the most lethal nosocomial infection, and overall it is the most frequent cause of death in developing countries. The incidence of pneumonia is high among infants and toddlers, declines greatly in childhood, remains relatively uncommon among young adults, but begins to increase after 50 years of age and especially after 65 years of age. About 3% of persons over 65 years of age in the USA are likely to develop pneumonia each year, of whom nearly one-half will be hospitalized, resulting in more than 1.5 million hospitalizations annually [7].

Not only is pneumonia more prevalent in elderly patients, it is also more severe, with the risk for death rising steadily with increasing age. Overall, about 7% of patients hospitalized for pneumonia die within 7 days, and another 7% die in the ensuing 30 days.

Pneumonia is an infection that involves a complex set of steps, beginning with initial contact with a pathogenic microorganism and culminating in the invasion of the lower respiratory tract. This infection can be acquired in the community or within the hospital setting, and can be transmitted by aspirated or inhaled microorganisms.

Pneumonia is a severe health problem and a significant cause of mortality and morbidity worldwide. In 2013, pneumonia was the eighth most common cause of death in the USA. In the USA alone it is responsible for approximately 1.1 million hospital admissions, 50,000 deaths, and close to 14,000 hospital readmissions per year. Pneumonia can be bacterial, viral, or fungal (but most commonly bacterial). It is important to understand the role of the different pathogens in the microbial etiology of pneumonia to effectively manage and guide appropriate antibiotic therapy. This handbook will focus on bacterial pneumonia and will cover the most clinically relevant information, including important features of pneumonia, microbial etiology, clinical course, diagnostic testing, management issues, and antimicrobial treatment and prevention [8].

5.4 Causes

Bacterial pneumonia generally does not affect healthy young adults, rather most adults, of any age, who develop bacterial pneumonia are likely to have one or more underlying predisposing conditions.

Most common is an antecedent viral respiratory infection, which increases adherence of bacteria to respiratory epithelial cells and damages clearance mechanisms by interfering with ciliary action. Influenza virus infection greatly increases the susceptibility to pneumonia caused by *Staphylococcus aureus, Streptococcus pneumoniae*, or *Haemophilus influenzae* and recent studies have confirmed that most of the deaths attributed to influenza virus during the great pandemic of 1918–1919 were due to bacterial superinfection.

Other viral respiratory infections, even if severe, appear to be less likely to predispose to bacterial pneumonia.

Chronic obstructive pulmonary disease (COPD; cystic fibrosis, and bronchiectasis or other structural abnormalities of the lung greatly predispose to bacterial pneumonia, especially in patients who are also taking corticosteroids. Other predisposing factors include cigarette smoking, which increases pulmonary secretions and damages ciliary action; malnutrition, which weakens the immune system; excessive alcohol intake, which suppresses the cough reflex and affects migration of white blood cells (WBCs); hepatic or renal disease, both of which decrease antibody formation and WBC function; diabetes mellitus, which decreases WBC function; and immunoglobulin deficiencies of any cause.

The nearly 100-fold increase in bacterial pneumonia in young adults who have AIDS is thought to be related largely to defective antibody production.

Factors predisposing older adults to pneumonia include diminished gag and cough reflexes, poor glottal function, and diminished toll-like receptor and antibody responses. These factors are far more prominent in persons who are frail or bedridden—whether at home, in a nursing facility, or in a hospital—than they are in healthy aging persons.

In contrast to bacterial pneumonia, viral or mycoplasmal pneumonia may occur at any age when organisms are transmitted to immunologically naïve hosts. The presence or absence of preexisting immunity and the general competence of the immune system itself appear to be principal determinants of whether infection occurs. Immune compromise contributes greatly to the severity of pneumonia due to respiratory syncytial virus, influenza virus, and parainfluenza virus, whereas pregnancy predisposes to severe influenza pneumonia.

Polymerase chain reaction (PCR) technology can identify respiratory viruses alone or together with a potential bacterial cause in 20–30% of patients hospitalized for pneumonia. Depending upon the season and year, influenza may be the most common, followed by respiratory syncytial virus and human metapneumovirus. Finding evidence for a viral infection by PCR does not exclude the possibility that a secondary bacterial infection is also present (Tables 5.1 and 5.2).

Table 5.1 Nagaratnam et al. [2]

Anatomical changes	Physiological changes	Effects in respiratory function
I. Changes in thoracic cage		
(i) Calcification of the intercostal cartilages; arthritis of the costa-vertebral joints	Rigidity and stiffness of the wall increases and chest wall compliance decreases	Expiratory flow movement decreases/shifts chest wall pressure-volume curve to the right
(ii) Gradual atrophy of intercostals muscles (loss of muscle mass)	Weakening of the intercostals muscles	Reduction in the muscle strength demands greater contribution from diaphragmatic and abdominal muscles and may lead to diaphragmatic fatigue
II. Airway changes		
(i) The cilia beat decreases with age and there is a reduction in number of cilia	Reduces clearance of debris and pathogens	Increases chance of infection
(ii) The conduction zone (the, area between nose and bronchioles) increases in size of the larger airways—trachea, Iry and II ry bronchi	Increase in volume of anatomical dead space	Increased residual volume and functional residual capacity and decreased vital capacity
(iii) Bronchioles and alveolar ducts increase in size, grouping of the alveoli, widening and loss of depth and loss of supporting tissue (`senile emphysema')	Decreased state of elastic recoil	Increased ventilation/perfusion heterogeneity
(iv) Thickening of the alveolar basement membrane	Decrease gas-diffusing capabilities, increase in ventilation/perfusion heterogeneity	Arterial oxygenation declines, CO transfer decreases
(v) Decrease in small airways diameter	Decrease in maxima] expiratory flow	Obstructive flow pattern
III. Ventilation control	Dimi rushes	Diminishes response to hypercapnia and hypoxia

Table 5.2 Modified table from 2 [6]

Underlying condition	Associated microorganism (Goldman [6])
Aspiration/poor dentition	Microaerophilic and anaerobic mouth flora
Gross aspiration, bedridden person	*Staphylococcus aureus,* gram-negative rods, microaerophilic and anaerobic mouth flora
Travel to southwestern United States	*Coccidioides immitis*
Residence in Mississippi River basins, exposure to bats	*Histoplasma capsulatum*
Exposure to birds	*Cryptococcus neoformans, H. capsulatum*
Exposure to sick psittacine birds	*Chlamydia psittaci*

(continued)

Table 5.2 (continued)

Exposure to rabbits	*Francisella tularensis*
Exposure to farm animals	*Coxiella burnetii* (Q fever)
Influenza active in community	Influenza virus, *S. aureus, S. pneumoniae, H. influenzae, Streptococcus pyogenes*
Bronchiectasis, cystic fibrosis	*Pseudomonas aeruginosa, Burkholderia cepacia, S. aureus, Aspergillus* species, nontuberculous mycobacteria
Cavitary lung lesion	Microaerophilic and anaerobic mouth flora, *S. aureus,* tuberculous and nontuberculous mycobacteria, endemic fungi
Intravenous drug use	*S. aureus, M. tuberculosis, S. pneumoniae*
Endobronchial obstruction	Microaerophilic and anaerobic mouth flora, gram-negative bacilli, *S. aureus*
Recent antibiotic therapy	Antibiotic-resistant *S. pneumoniae*
HIV (early)	*S. pneumoniae, H. influenzae, M. tuberculosis*
HIV/AIDS	Pathogens listed for early HIV infection, plus *Pneumocystis jirovecii, Cryptococcus, Histoplasma, Aspergillus, Mycobacterium kansasii, Mycobacterium avium* complex, *P. aeruginosa*
Travel to Middle East and 2019–2020 China	Middle East respiratory syndrome (MERS) , SARS, and SARS-COV2
Bioterrorism	*Bacillus anthracis* (anthrax), *Yersinia pestis* (plague), *Francisella tularensis* (tularemia)

5.5 Routes of Transmission

Pathogens that cause pneumonia can reach the lower respiratory tract by any of four mechanisms: inhalation, aspiration, hematogenous spread, or direct extension from adjacent foci, as detailed below (Fig. 5.1 from [8]).

5.5.1 Inhalation (Fig. 5.1)

Inhalation is the most common route of infection in community-acquired cases of pneumonia in younger healthy patients (Fig. 5.1 from [8]).

Viral and atypical pneumonia also usually develops via this route of transmission. Aerosol (droplet nuclei) transmission occurs when water and pathogen-laden respiratory droplets are exhaled by an infected person, desiccate so that they become light enough to remain suspended in the air for minutes to hours, and are then inhaled into the respiratory tract of a susceptible person to initiate infection. In the case of droplet spray transmission, an infected person coughs or sneezes, expelling respiratory droplets containing contagious particles, which impact directly on the nasal mucosa of a susceptible person. Inhalation pneumonia develops when pathogens bypass the respiratory defense mechanisms or when the patient inhales aerobic Gram-negative pathogens that colonize the upper respiratory tract or respiratory support equipment. In HAP this occurs with pathogens such as *Legionella pneumophila, Mycobacterium tuberculosis,* and respiratory viruses: Influenza virus, Coronavirus: COVID-19 (sars-cov 2), mers, sars.

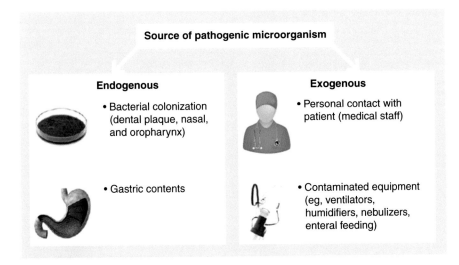

Fig. 5.1   Sources of pathogenic microorganisms associated with pneumonia

5.5.2   Aspiration (Fig. 5.2)

Aspiration of oropharyngeal secretions into the trachea is the primary route through which pathogens enter into the lower airways (Fig. 5.2 from [8]).

In the community, nasopharyngeal carriage rates of pneumococcus in healthy children and adults ranges from 20% to 50% and 5% to 30%, respectively [4, 5]. In a healthy, nonimmune person, previous viral infections can facilitate the transfer of pneumococcus from the oropharynx to the lower respiratory tract. The oropharynx of hospitalized patients is colonized with Gram-negative pathogens in 35–75% of patients within 3–5 days of admission, depending on the severity and type of underlying illness. Risk factors for CAP pathogens include prior antibiotic treatment, length of hospitalization, intubation, smoking, alcohol consumption, malnutrition, and dental plaque. Ewig et al. found that the initial colonization rate of any site (nasal and pharyngeal, tracheobronchial, and gastric juice) following intensive care unit (ICU) admission for brain injury was 83%. *Streptococcus pneumoniae, Haemophilus influenzae,* and *Staphylococcus aureus* were the predominant pathogens identified in the upper airways.

5.5.3   Hematogenous Spread (Fig. 5.3)

Pneumonia can be acquired by hematogenous spread of pathogens from another site of infection (e.g., endocarditis) to the lungs, although this route of transmission is rare. Pneumonia due to hematogenous spread of *S. aureus* is a unique type of pneumonia, usually occurring as a consequence of intravenous drug abuse or septic

Fig. 5.2 Pathogenic bacteria present in oropharyngeal secretions enter the lower respiratory tract by transport through the trachea, facilitating disease in sensitive and immunosuppressed hosts: Aspiration pneumonia

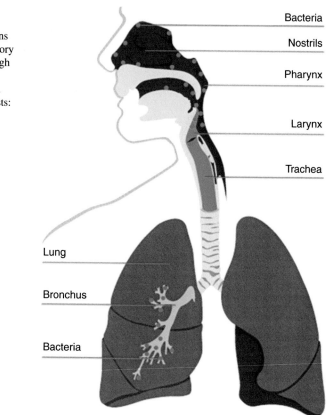

embolization from endocarditis or an infected vascular site. In cases acquired hematogenously, signs and symptoms related to the underlying endovascular infection predominate; if pulmonary infarction results from a septic embolism, pleuritic chest pain and hemoptysis are often noted (Fig. 5.3 from [8]).

Hematogenous pneumonia presents with bilateral symmetrical perihilar infiltrates, as opposed to the localized segmental or lobar distribution characteristic of pneumonia acquired via primary inhalation.

5.5.4 Direct Extension from Adjacent Infected Foci (Fig. 5.4)

Microbial pathogens may enter the lung by direct spread from a contiguous site of infection (Fig. 5.4 from [8]).

For example, tuberculosis can spread contiguously from lymph nodes to the pericardium or the lung, but this is rarely a mode of transmission for pneumonia.

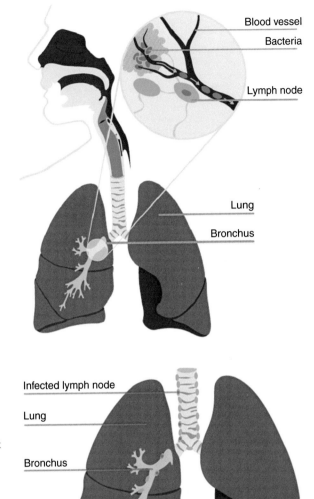

Fig. 5.3 Pneumonia can be acquired by the spread of pathogens into the lung from another infected site (e.g., endocarditis, pyelonephritis, peritonitis) by blood transport, although this route of transmission is rare: Hematogenic diffusion

Fig. 5.4 Pathogens such as in tuberculosis can cause disease by spreading directly to the lung from another infection site; however, this is rare: Direct extension from adjacent foci

5.6   Clinical Presentation

Pneumonia in elderly patients was described by William Osler as a painless and fatal disease. The disease was described as latent, without chills, with mild cough, and sometimes without sputum.

Physical examination was marked owing to the lack of classic evidence of consolidation, and mental status changes might be the only sign of pneumonia.

Not much has changed in our knowledge regarding pneumonia manifestations in the elderly. Fever may be absent in 25–55% of pneumonia cases in older adults, and a similar proportion of elderly patients present with altered mental status.

Of 48 patients older than 65 years in a veteran's administration medical center who were diagnosed with pneumonia based on new pulmonary infiltrates and symptoms, only 35% presented with fever and cough.

The absence of classic symptoms was more common in patients with reduced baseline functional capacity.

A study that evaluated 1812 patients from four US hospitals demonstrated that, as patients became older, the number of reported symptoms of pneumonia decreased.

Among patients who reside in LTCFs, pneumonia-related signs and symptoms were demonstrated to be subtler than in CAP patients from the same age group. As many as 73% of these LTCF cases present with confusion. Fever and respiratory symptoms were less common than in other CAP patients.

In residents of LTCFs, diagnosis of pneumonia based on symptoms and physical examination has low sensitivity and specificity (47–69% and 58–75%, respectively).

In addition, owing to the presence of other comorbid conditions, there is often a broad and nonspecific differential diagnosis, which can lead to diagnostic challenges and delays. An association between latent pneumonia and poor outcomes was described by Osler William, who stressed that fever may actually be a positive predictor of outcome, a notion that was later supported by other researchers.

The diagnosis of pneumonia in the elderly depends on a high index of suspicion and should be considered in the presence of one of the following atypical signs and symptoms: confusion, delirium, disorientation, or loss of appetite. Particularly in an older adult with dementia, urinary incontinence may sometimes be an early indicator of debility caused by pneumonia. These atypical symptoms should not be automatically attributed to a patient's baseline dementia. Unexplained deterioration in general health, weakness, new onset of recurrent falls, and functional decline (i.e., general deterioration) may also be important manifestations of pneumonia in older adults, as well as exacerbation of underlying illnesses, such as congestive heart failure, chronic pulmonary lung disease, and impaired diabetic control [9].

Simple physical examination findings, including respiratory rate (>25 breathes/min) and pulse oximetry (oxygen saturation < 90%), have a high sensitivity for pneumonia and, if present, indicate the need for further evaluation of pneumonia, potentially including imaging, testing, and referral to an acute care hospital.

In bacterial pneumonia, crackles or rales are generally present over the affected area. Bronchial breath sounds and egophony strongly suggest pneumonia when present but are not sensitive for diagnosis. Dullness to percussion over the affected area may be detected in about one-half of cases. Increased tactile fremitus is often present and is especially useful in distinguishing a pulmonary infiltrate from a pleural effusion, in which fremitus is diminished or absent. The failure to detect excursion of the diaphragm by percussion suggests an effusion. Unfortunately, the overall sensitivity and specificity of the physical examination for pneumonia is fairly low, perhaps related to inadequate training. In all cases, the diagnosis of pneumonia requires radiographic validation.

In one study of LTFC subjects with pneumonia, an oxygen saturation of less than 94% was sensitive and specific for the diagnosis of pneumonia (80% and 91%, respectively).

The respiratory rate may be increased; a rate of more than 25 breaths/min should cause serious concern. An oxygen saturation (SaO_2) of less than 92% is likely to indicate a very low partial pressure of oxygen in arterial blood, and a low saturation together with a rapid respiratory rate suggests serious respiratory compromise with impending respiratory distress [10].

The clinical presentation of COVID-19 can be indistinguishable from other viral causes of pneumonia and include:

- Fever (83–99%)
- Cough (59–82%)
- Fatigue (44–70%)
- Anorexia (40–84%)
- Shortness of breath (31–40%)
- Sputum production (28–33%)
- Myalgia (11–35%)

Older adults and persons with medical comorbidities may have delayed presentation of fever and respiratory symptoms, scarce or silent semeiological picture in front of an important radiological picture with diffuse non-focal peribronchiolar interstitial involvement. Dyspnoea, hypocapnic hypoxemia, non-leukocytosis, lymphopenia [11].

COVID-19 is a sneaky disease that has surprised many medical experts.

In one study of 1099 hospitalized patients, fever was present in only 44% at hospital admission but later developed in 89% during hospitalization.

Headache, confusion, rhinorrhea, sore throat, hemoptysis, vomiting, and diarrhea have been reported but are less common (<10%). Some persons with COVID-19 have experienced gastrointestinal symptoms such as diarrhea and nausea prior to developing fever and lower respiratory tract signs and symptoms.

Anosmia or ageusia preceding the onset of respiratory symptoms has been anecdotally reported, but more information is needed to understand its role in identifying COVID-19. The median age of confirmed COVID-19 cases is in the sixth decade of life with a slight male predominance.

Twenty-five percent of patients have severe symptoms requiring intensive care treatment of which 10% develop respiratory failure requiring mechanical ventilation. Chest radiograph imaging of these patients reveals bilateral patchy infiltrates and CT imaging shows ground-glass infiltrates. Patients typically present with laboratory findings of prolonged prothrombin time, elevated lactate dehydrogenase, and lymphopenia (70% of patients). However, it is unclear if the lymphopenia is related to direct cytotoxic effect of the virus or underlying chronic conditions [12].

5.7 COVID-19 Pneumonia "Phenotypes"

A controversial report suggested that COVID-19 patients appear to have at least two phenotypes, from the perspective of ICU management [13].

However, this classification is largely based on anecdote, remains preliminary, and management should be optimized for each individual patient as clinically indicated.

5.7.1 L-Phenotype

- Typical of early presentation viral pneumonitis
- Hypoxemia with preserved CO_2 clearance (Type 1 respiratory failure)
- Low Elastance (i.e., high compliance)
- Low V/Q matching (possibly due to abnormal hypoxic vasoconstriction)
- Low Recruitability (poor response to PEEP and proning)
- Implications: May be able to avoid mechanical ventilation with appropriate oxygen therapy. May be responsive to pulmonary vasodilators (e.g., inhaled nitric oxide)

5.7.2 H-Phenotype

Typical of later illness and classic ARDS, including patients who have had prolonged noninvasive ventilation (potential for patient-induced lung injury from volutrauma and barotrauma) and coexisting lung disease or complications:

- Hypoxemia +/– impaired CO2 clearance (Type 1 and/or 2 respiratory failure)
- High Elastance (i.e., low compliance)
- High V/Q matching
- High Recruitability (response to PEEP and proning)

Implications: May benefit from protective lung ventilation and usual ARDS therapies (potentially including an "open lung approach").

The existence and utility of these phenotypes is being increasingly called into question as observed cohorts suggest that COVID-19 presentations are consistent with prior descriptions of ARDS [14].

5.8 Risk Stratification

Severity-of-illness scores or prognostic models, such as the CURB-65 criteria or the Pneumonia Severity Index (PSI) can be used to help identify patients that may be candidates for outpatient treatment and those that may require admission (see below). The Infectious Disease Society of America (IDSA) and American Thoracic Society (ATS) proposed guidelines and criteria to determine the severity of community-acquired pneumonia (CAP), which would affect whether inpatient treatment would occur on the ward or require ICU care [15].

Although many of these predictive models were originally designed for assessment of CAP, a retrospective cohort study determined that they may also be applicable to HCAP [16].

5.8.1   CURB-65 (Table 5.3)

CURB-65 is a scoring system developed from a multivariate analysis of 1068 patients that identified various factors that appeared to play a role in patient mortality (Table 5.3). One point is given for the presence of each of the following:

- **C** onfusion—Altered mental status
- **U** remia—Blood urea nitrogen (BUN) level greater than 20 mg/dL
- **R** espiratory rate—30 breaths or more/min
- **B** lood pressure—Systolic pressure less than 90 mmHg or diastolic pressure less than 60 mmHg
- **A** ge older than 65 years

Current guidelines suggest that patients may be treated in an outpatient setting or may require hospitalization according to their CURB-65 score, as follows:

- Score of 0–1—Outpatient treatment
- Score of 2—Admission to medical ward
- Score of 3 or higher—Admission to intensive care unit (ICU)

The percentage of mortality at 30 days associated with the various CURB-65 scores increases with higher scores. The drastic increase in mortality between scores of two and three highlights the likely requirement for ICU admission in patients with a score of three or higher, as shown below:

- Score of 0–0.7% mortality
- Score of 1–2.1% mortality
- Score of 2–9.2% mortality

Table 5.3 The CURB-65 scores range from 0 to 5. Assign points as in the table based on confusion status, urea level, respiratory rate, blood pressure, and age [15]

	POINTS
Confusion	1
Elevated blood **U**rea nitrogen	1
Respiratory rate ≥30/min	1
Low **B**lood pressure (hypotension)	1
Age ≥ **65** years	1

Assign 1 point each for each of the 5 features listed above. Hospital admission is recommended for patients with 2 or more points and intensive care admission for 3 or more ponits.

- Score of 3–14.5% mortality
- Score of 4–40% mortality
- Score of 5–57% mortality

5.8.2 Pneumonia Severity Index, Also Known as the PORT Score
(Fig. 5.5 and Table 5.4)

The PSI, also known as the PORT score (for the study by which it was validated), is a prediction rule for mortality based on characteristics derived from cohorts of patients hospitalized with pneumonia [17].

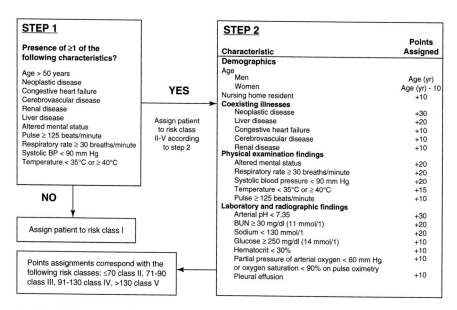

Fig. 5.5 PSI Points are assigned based on age, comorbid disease, abnormal physical findings, and abnormal laboratory results

Table 5.4 Port severity index (PSI) and mortality at 30 days [17]

POINT SCORE	CLASS	MORTALITY		
		COMMUNITY-ACQUIRED PNEUMONIA	COMMUNITY-ACQUIRED PNEUMONIA	PNEUMOCOCCAL PNEUMONIA
≤70	II	<1%	3%	—
71-90	III	3%	4%	3%
91-130	IV	8%	8%	21%
>130	V	29%	22%	35%

For each of the various characteristics, a predetermined value of points is assigned. In a retrospective cohort comparison of different predictive models applied to HCAP, the PSI had the highest sensitivity in predicting mortality. However, alternative tools, including the IDSA/ATS, SCAP, and SMART-COP (mentioned below), are considered easier to calculate.

When a pneumonia is due to mixed etiologies, it is often underestimated by severity scores [18, 19].

By comparing the PSI scores with CURB-65, it was shown that CURB-65 offers the same sensitivity as the prediction of mortality due to community-acquired pneumonia. In particular, CURB-65 (74.6%) has a specificity higher than PSI (52.2%). However, CURB-65 had a lower sensitivity than PSI in predicting ICU admission.

5.8.3   IDSA/ATS CAP Criteria

Prediction rules like the CURB-65 and PSI have proven useful for standardizing clinical assessments and identifying low-risk patients who may be appropriate candidates for outpatient therapy, but they have been less useful for discriminating between moderate (ward-appropriate) and high-risk (ICU-appropriate) patients. The IDSA/ATS criteria for severe community-acquired pneumonia (CAP) are composed of both major and minor criteria. Although the major criteria indicate clear need for ICU-level care, the minor criteria for defining severe CAP have been validated for the use of differentiating between patients requiring ward-level versus ICU-level care [20]. These criteria are particularly helpful in identifying those patients who are appropriate for admission to the ICU but who do not meet the major criteria of requiring mechanical ventilation or vasopressor support.

The presence of three of the following minor criteria indicates severe CAP and suggests the likely need for ICU-level care:

- Respiratory rate of 30 breaths or more/min
- Ratio of PaO_2 to fraction of inspired oxygen (i.e., PaO_2/FiO_2) of 250 or less
- Need for noninvasive ventilation (bilevel positive airway pressure [BiPAP] or continuous positive airway pressure [CPAP])
- Multilobar infiltrates
- Confusion/disorientation
- Uremia (BUN 20 mg/dL or greater)
- Leukopenia (white blood cell [WBC] count less than 4000 cells/μL)
- Thrombocytopenia (platelet count less than 100,000/μL)
- Hypothermia (core temperature less than 36 °C)
- Hypotension requiring aggressive fluid resuscitation

The major criteria are as follows:

- Invasive mechanical ventilation
- Septic shock requiring vasopressor support

Table. 5.5 SMART-COP Score for Pneumonia Severity

	POINTS
Low **S**ystolic blood pressure (<90 mm Hg)	2
Multilobar involvement (on chest radiograph)	1
Low **A**lbumin (<3.5 g/dL)	1
High **R**espiratory rate (≥25 if <50 years old, ≥30 if >50 years old)	1
Tachycardia (heart rate >125 beats/min)	1
New-onset **C**onfusion	1
Poor **O**xygenation (Pao$_2$ <70 mm Hg if <50 years old, <60 mm Hg if >50 years old	2
Low arterial **pH** (<7.35)	2

Direct admission to an ICU is mandated for any patient with septic shock and a requirement for intravenous vasopressors support or with acute respiratory failure requiring intubation and mechanical ventilation.

Multiple other scoring models exist that can be used to aid in the prediction of mortality in severe illness (namely in the ICU setting), including the acute physiology and chronic health evaluation (APACHE II) score, simplified acute physiology score (SAPS II), and sepsis-related organ failure assessment (SOFA) score.

Whereas most scoring models have been used for predicting outcomes in patients carrying a diagnosis of CAP, the systolic blood pressure, oxygenation, age, respiratory rate (SOAR) model has been validated for predicting 30-day mortality in patients hospitalized with nursing home-acquired pneumonia (NHAP). Still other prediction models regarding pneumonia severity and outcomes are currently being explored and developed, such as the Spanish CURXO-80 tool; predisposition, insult, response, and organ dysfunction (PIRO) tool; and systolic blood pressure, multilobar involvement, albumin level, respiratory rate, tachycardia, confusion, oxygenation and arterial pH (SMART-COP) tool (Table 5.5).

With the start of the SARS-COV 2 pandemic, further specific scores have been conceived:

5.8.4 COVID-GRAM Critical Illness Risk Score

Predict occurrence of ICU admission, mechanical ventilation, or death in hospitalized patients with COVID-19 (https://www.mdcalc.com/covid-gram-critical-illness-risk-score#evidence). Early identification of patients with COVID-19 who may develop critical illness is important to aid in delivering proper treatment and optimize use of limited resources. The COVID–GRAM predictive risk score was developed in collaboration with the National Health Commission of China from a retrospective cohort of patients diagnosed with COVID-19 before January 31, 2020.

Epidemiological, clinical, laboratory, and imaging data were collected from 575 hospitals in 31 provincial administrative regions in China.

Ten variables at the time of admission were identified to be independently statistically significant predictors of critical illness:

– Age
– Unconsciousness
– Hemoptysis
– Dyspnea
– Number of comorbidities
– Cancer history
– CXR abnormality
– Neutrophil-to-lymphocyte ratio
– Lactate dehydrogenase
– Direct bilirubin

• The risk score was validated with data from four additional cohorts hospitalized in China with COVID-19. It estimates the risk of developing critical illness (defined as requiring ICU admission, mechanical ventilation, or death). The accuracy of the risk score was assessed using the area under the receiver-operator characteristic curve (AUC). Based on data from the development cohort, the accuracy of the risk score was 0.88 (95% CI, 0.85–0.91). The AUC for patients in the epicenter at Hubei was 0.87 (95% CI, 0.83–0.91) and outside Hubei was 0.82 (95% CI, 0.73–0.90). CURB-6 models, which have been used to classify the severity of community-acquired pneumonia, had an AUC of 0.75 (95% CI, 0.70–0.80) comparatively [21].

5.8.5 Brescia-COVID Respiratory Severity Scale (BCRSS)/ Algorithm

Stepwise management approach to COVID-19 patients based on clinical severity as of March 27, 2020. This algorithm is a stepwise approach to managing patients with confirmed/presumed COVID-19 pneumonia. If not intubated, follow management and then each four testing criteria should be repeated to assess for improvement or deterioration. Repetition frequency is based on clinical judgment to downgrade/upgrade score. Not only is the management important, but the numerical score is also used to easily compare and summarize patients to treating clinicians. NIV is concerning for aerosolization, but it is included in score due to ventilator scarcity in Italy (https://cdn-web-img.mdcalc.com/content/BRSS_A4.pdf).
• *Neutrophil-Lymphocyte Ratio (NLR) Calculator*: Calculates neutrophil-lymphocyte ratio (https://www.ncbi.nlm.nih.gov/pmc/articles/PMC7152924/).

5.9 Imaging

Evaluating imaging findings in elderly persons with suspected pneumonia is challenging. The classic pulmonary opacity used as part of the gold standard for diagnosis of pneumonia may not be identified by a regular chest radiograph owing to poor film quality (Fig. 5.6).

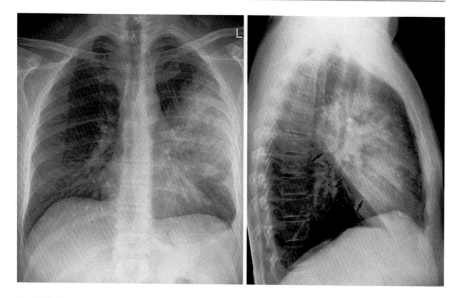

Fig. 5.6 Lobar pneumonia—Radiological staff archive Dr. Attilio De Blasio

Pneumonia is diagnosed by the presence of an infiltrate on chest imaging or excluded by its absence. Detection of radiographic infiltrates can be surprisingly difficult, especially in patients who have chronic lung disease, are obese, or are evaluated with only a portable chest radiograph.

Small areas of alveolar consolidation may be missed by a chest radiograph, especially an anterior-posterior radiograph taken at the patient's bedside, but be detected by the far more sensitive computed tomography (CT) scan. CT may also demonstrate that seeming abnormalities on plain chest radiography are false positives. However, small areas of apparent consolidation ("ground-glass changes") are often described on the CT scan of patients who do not have pneumonia. Bedside ultrasonography may also be used to detect pulmonary infiltrates, but its sensitivity and specificity, though relatively high [3], are not sufficient to obviate the need for a chest radiograph. Up to 40% of patients with pneumonia also have a parapneumonic effusion that is detectable by special studies (Fig. 5.7).

Although the presence of a newly recognized pulmonary infiltrate is the sine qua non of diagnosing pneumonia, the radiographic appearance provides very little insight into the etiology. Dense consolidation of a segment or lobe is usually bacterial, especially due to *S. pneumoniae* or *Klebsiella*. Other bacteria, including *Legionella*, may cause a similar picture, but many bacterial pneumonias cause subsegmental infiltrates. Viral pneumonia does not cause segmental or lobar consolidation.

Pneumonia due to microaspiration of *S. aureus* or gram-negative bacilli cannot be distinguished radiographically from other bacterial pneumonias. Although these are said to be more likely to cavitate, that conclusion may reflect reporting bias. Pneumococcal pneumonia also causes lung necrosis that is visible on a chest radiograph in 2% of cases and on CT in 11% of cases.

Fig. 5.7 Lobar pneumonia
in CT scan of the thorax—
Radiological staff archive
dott. Attilio De Blasio

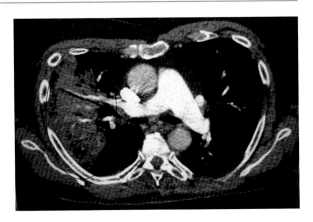

One of the few radiologically distinctive bacterial pneumonia is that due to hematogenous spread of *S. aureus*, especially when it occurs with endocarditis or an infected intravascular source. Hematogenous *S. aureus* pneumonia causes 1- to 3-cm round lesions, which are likely to cavitate. Subsegmental or "patchy" pneumonia may be due to bacteria, viruses, *Mycoplasma,* or *Chlamydia. Pneumocystis jirovecii* causes a diffuse interstitial infiltrate that may, in its earlier clinical stages, be mistaken for prominent pulmonary markings. Aspiration of mixed anaerobic, microaerophilic, and facultative bacteria from the mouth may cause pneumonia but may also lead to a lung abscess with a thick wall, a fluid level, and surrounding consolidation, especially in the superior segments of the lower lobes or posterior segments of the upper lobes. A cavitary lesion of an upper lobe without a fluid level, especially if confined to the posterior segment, suggests tuberculosis, a nontuberculous *Mycobacterium,* or nocardiosis. Occasionally, more acute presentations of tuberculosis may mimic acute bacterial pneumonia. *Aspergillus* can proliferate within a cavity to cause the distinctive appearance of an intracavitary mycetoma (fungus ball) surrounded by an arc or halo of air [10].

Rapidly progressive pneumonia of any cause may result in diffuse pulmonary infiltrates consistent with the acute respiratory distress syndrome or diffuse alveolar hemorrhage. Although the appearance or enlargement of infiltrates after patients are hospitalized and treatment is begun is often attributed to fluid repletion, such progression more likely reflects the ongoing inflammatory response. A chest CT scan may help clarify the nature of an infiltrate and will determine whether an effusion or mass is present, but it is usually not necessary at hospital admission for patients in whom a good-quality chest radiograph can be obtained.

Poor quality might be owing in part to the patient's poor cognitive status, poor muscle strength, and inability to maintain posture. In addition, lung disease (chronic obstructive pulmonary disease, malignancies, interstitial lung disease) and chest wall abnormalities, which are more frequent in the elderly, may complicate the interpretation of chest radiographs. In several studies of elderly patients, computed tomography (CT) scan detected pneumonia in up to 47% of cases that were not identified by using chest radiographs [22].

There are also interobserver discrepancies in the interpretation of chest radiographs, which may be particularly problematic when portable chest radiographs are used.

Among residents of LTCFs, imaging has an important role in the diagnosis of pneumonia, as well as in identifying other high-risk conditions that warrant the transfer to an acute care facility. Often, LTCFs have contracted services that provide portable chest radiographs; these portable chest radiographs have similar limitations to standard chest radiographs, as described. Further complicating the usefulness of chest radiographs in LTCFs is a lack of previous films for comparison.

Nevertheless, several studies have reported that 75–90% of chest radiographs taken for evaluation of suspected pneumonia among LTCF residents showed evidence of pneumonia. Thus, chest radiograph should be conducted as part of the evaluation of pneumonia in LTCF residents.

Although CT scan is the gold standard for diagnosis of pneumonia, limitations such as cost, radiation exposure, availability, and identification of incidental findings, which are particularly common in the elderly, limit its usefulness. Chest CT should be limited to cases where chest radiograph findings are inconclusive, pneumonia complications might be present (e.g., lung abscess), or when there is suspicion for pathologies that cannot be diagnosed by chest radiograph (e.g., pulmonary embolism, tumor). Evaluating imaging findings in elderly persons with suspected pneumonia is challenging. The classic pulmonary opacity used as part of the gold standard for diagnosis of pneumonia may not be identified by a regular chest radiograph owing to poor film quality [23]. Pneumonia is diagnosed by the presence of an infiltrate on chest imaging or excluded by its absence. Detection of radiographic infiltrates can be surprisingly difficult, especially in patients who have chronic lung disease, are obese, or are evaluated with only a portable chest radiograph. Several studies have demonstrated a lack of agreement in the interpretation of chest radiographs bringing their role as the ultimate arbiter of diagnosis of pneumonia. In fact, small areas of alveolar consolidation may be missed by a chest radiograph, especially an anterior-posterior radiograph taken at the patient's bedside, but be detected by the far more sensitive computed tomography (CT) scan. CT may also demonstrate that seeming abnormalities on plain chest radiography are false positives. However, small areas of apparent consolidation ("ground-glass changes") are often described on the CT scan of patients who do not have pneumonia.

Furthermore, COVID-19 pneumonia manifests with chest CT imaging abnormalities, even in asymptomatic patients, with rapid evolution from focal unilateral to diffuse bilateral ground-glass opacities that progressed to or coexisted with consolidations within 1–3 weeks (Fig. 5.8).

Lung ultrasound (LUS) imaging was recently evaluated for the diagnosis of CAP in the elderly, when the chest radiograph findings were inconclusive. In a cohort of 169 elderly frail patients, the sensitivity of LUS imaging was 91% and of chest radiograph was 47% (gold standard was considered to be clinical diagnosis, with or without CT scan). Recent meta-analyses that evaluated LUS imaging for the diagnosis of pneumonia reported a pooled sensitivity of 94–95% and specificity of 90–96% when LUS imaging findings were compared with diagnosis of pneumonia by clinical signs and/or chest radiograph or CT findings, and a high correlation

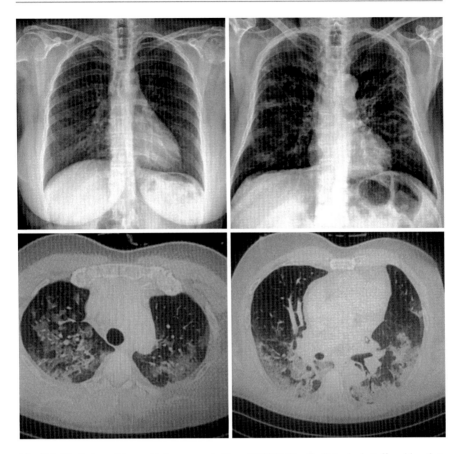

Fig. 5.8 Evolution of interstitial pneumonia from COVID-19—Radiological staff archive dott. Attilio De Blasio

between LUS imaging and CT findings was reported (Spearman correlation coefficient of 0.87) [24, 25].

Radiographic resolution lags behind clinical resolution of pneumonia, but older age was not found to be associated with delayed resolution compared with younger age groups [26].

5.10 Laboratory Investigations

Most patients with bacterial pneumonia have a WBC count higher than 11,000/μL at the time of admission to hospital, and about one-third have a WBC count higher than 15,000 WBC/μL.

A normal WBC count should not be interpreted as reassuring because WBC counts of 6000/μL or less may be seen in overwhelming bacterial infection. When overwhelming bacterial infection suppresses the WBC count, immature (band) cells are almost always elevated. Nevertheless, WBC counts higher than 20,000/μL are unusual in acute pulmonary conditions other than bacterial pneumonia. Mild nonspecific elevations in the serum bilirubin level, aminotransferase levels, and lactate dehydrogenase (LDH) level are often noted. Marked elevations of the LDH level can be seen in Pneumocystis pneumonia and in disseminated Histoplasma infection in AIDS patients.

An elevated serum procalcitonin level increases the likelihood of a bacterial infection, but a low level is not sufficiently sensitive to exclude such a diagnosis. Although some randomized trials of patients who present with lower respiratory tract symptoms suggested that a treatment guided by the procalcitonin level (antibiotics discouraged if the level is ≤0.25 µg/L and strongly discouraged if <0.1 µg/L) could safely reduce antibiotic usage, the most recent U.S. trial found no benefit in hospitals with high adherence to guidelines for treating pneumonia.

Furthermore, 25% of patients with bacterial pneumonia have a normal procalcitonin level, and up to 25% of patients with a pneumonia syndrome but no evidence for bacterial infection have an elevated procalcitonin level, so this test cannot be used alone to determine therapeutic decisions.

5.11 Microbiologic Diagnosis

Sputum is composed of this exudate plasma, WBCs, and bacteria with a greater or lesser admixture of saliva. The presence of large numbers of a single type of bacterium (e.g., gram-positive cocci resembling pneumococci) in an inflammatory specimen that is relatively free of contaminating epithelial cells strongly suggests this organism as the etiologic agent of the pneumonia. In patients who have bacteremic pneumococcal pneumonia, who cough up a valid specimen, and who have not received antibiotics, microscopic examination of a gram-stained sputum is greater than 85% sensitive for detecting pneumococci and *H. influenzae* but may be lower for other bacteria. Because the sensitivity of Gram stain falls dramatically after 6 h, and that of culture, after 18 h of antibiotic treatment, specimens are useful diagnostically only if they are collected in a timely fashion.

Bacterial cultures will readily yield *Haemophilus, Moraxella, S. aureus*, or gram-negative bacilli when these organisms cause pneumonia. However, finding *S. aureus* or gram-negative rods by culture when they have not been seen microscopically in a good-quality sputum may suggest that these are contaminating mouth flora.

Enzyme-linked immunosorbent assay (ELISA) can detect pneumococcal cell wall or capsular polysaccharide in the urine of 60–80% of patients with bacteremic pneumococcal pneumonia and a smaller proportion of those with nonbacteremic disease; a urinary ELISA for specific pneumococcal serotypes is substantially more sensitive. An ELISA for urinary *Legionella* antigen detects only the most common *Legionella* serotype but is positive in about 70% of cases of *Legionella* pneumonia, with higher sensitivity in more severe disease. Histoplasma urine and Cryptococcus serum antigen tests are positive in patients with disseminated disease but are less likely to be positive in patients with discrete pulmonary infiltrates.

PCR testing of a nasopharyngeal specimen is a highly sensitive technique for detecting the presence of potentially infecting microorganisms, but a positive PCR may indicate colonization rather than infection. Quantitative PCR testing in African patients with AIDS and suspected pneumonia reliably identifies pneumococcal pneumonia, but the generalizability of this method to non-AIDS patients in developed countries remains to be determined. For organisms that do not normally colonize the upper airways, PCR is sensitive and specific. PCR on a throat swab can reliably detect *Chlamydia* and *Mycoplasma* as well as 15 respiratory viruses (including influenza, parainfluenza, respiratory syncytial virus, human metapneumovirus, coronavirus, and adenovirus) with very high sensitivity. These respiratory viruses are present in fewer than 2% of healthy adults, so the finding of a respiratory virus by PCR in a patient with pneumonia suggests an etiologic role. As a result, PCR has generally replaced viral culture as the gold standard for diagnosing influenza virus infection. It must be emphasized that finding evidence for a viral infection, especially due to influenza virus, does not preclude the possibility of a secondary bacterial infection. Sputum PCR also can detect *M. tuberculosis* and is now part of the recommended evaluation in patients suspected of having this diagnosis. Bacteremia is documented in 5–10% of patients who are hospitalized for community-acquired pneumonia, including 20–25% of patients with pneumococcal pneumonia, 10–15% of patients with aerogenous pneumonia due to *S. aureus* or gram-negative rods, a much lower proportion of patients with nontypable *H. influenzae* pneumonia, and only rarely in pneumonia caused by *Moraxella catarrhalis*. By comparison, patients with hematogenous *S. aureus* pneumonia virtually always have positive blood cultures. Pneumococcal pneumonia also can be diagnosed by the presence of serotype-specific urinary antigens.

Mycoplasma, Chlamydia, Coxiella burnetii, and *Legionella* are "atypical organisms." These organisms have in common their lack of typical cell walls. They also all respond to treatment with tetracyclines, macrolides, and quinolones. However, these infections have little else in common. Although *Mycoplasma* and *C. pneumoniae,* they cause fewer than 1–2% of cases that require hospitalization. Pneumonia caused by these organisms is characterized by prolonged nonproductive cough, low-grade fever, and scattered pulmonary infiltrates. PCR is preferred over serologies for diagnosing *Chlamydia* or *Mycoplasma* infections, because serologic studies substantially overestimate the prevalence of acute infection with these agents. Pneumonia due to *Legionella* behaves like a typical bacterial pneumonia and can often be traced to a water source, whereas pneumonia due to *C. burnetii* (Q fever) occurs late in summer and is associated with severe headache and elevation of liver enzymes [27].

5.12   Viral Aetiology (Fig. 5.9)

During an influenza outbreak, this virus is identified in a substantial proportion of patients admitted to intensive care for pneumonia. Identification of influenza virus in a patient with pneumonia should lead to appropriate antiviral treatment, even if more than 48 h have passed since the onset of symptoms. Secondary bacterial infection is common, with *S. aureus, S. pneumonia,* and *Haemophilus* predominating. Rhinovirus is the virus most commonly recognized in patients with pneumonia. Parainfluenza virus, respiratory syncytial virus, coronavirus SARS E SARS-COV2,

Virus	Nucleic Acid Type	Transmission	Seasonality in the United States	Prevention	Available Treatments
Influenza virus	RNA negative ss	Large, aerosolized droplets	Winter	Seasonal influenza vaccine	Oseltamivir, zanamivir amantadine
Rhinovirus	RNA positive ss	Aerosols, fomites	Throughout	Standard contact precautions	Symptomatic
Coronavirus (e.g., severe acute respiratory syndrome coronavirus, Middle East respiratory syndrome coronavirus)	RNA positive ss	Large aerosolized droplets, fomites	Spring and winter	Standard contact precautions	Symptomatic
Adenovirus	DNA double stranded	Aerosols, fomites	Throughout	Standard contact precautions, oral vaccine approved for U.S. military personnel only	Symptomatic; ribavirin can be used, but no proven clinical data to date
Human metapneumovirus	RNA negative ss	Large droplets, fomites	Spring and winter	Standard contact precautions	Symptomatic; cidofovir or ribavirin can be used, but no proven clinical data
Respiratory syncytial virus	RNA negative ss	Large droplets, fomites	Winter	Standard contact precautions	Symptomatic; ribavirin can be used in severe illness and immunocompromised patients
Parainfluenza virus	RNA negative ss	Large droplets, fomites	Throughout	Standard contact precautions	Symptomatic

ss = single stranded

Fig. 5.9 Classification of viral pneumonia

and human metapneumovirus are clearly implicated as causes of pneumonia in adults and elderly hospitalized for pneumonia and may require intensive care, so the severity of the lung involvement does not exclude the possibility that a viral infection alone is responsible. Outbreaks of adenovirus pneumonia occur in military recruits. Because coinfecting bacteria are also detected in 20–25% of cases of documented viral pneumonia, identifying a virus by PCR in a patient with pneumonia does not prove that the virus is the cause or especially the sole cause of illness. Other features, such as the history, severity of illness, sputum production (and, if present, microscopic examination), nature of the pulmonary infiltrate, WBC count, and procalcitonin level may help to clarify the etiologic diagnosis.

The clinical presentation of viral pneumonia does not differentiate between the specific viral causes of respiratory infection. The common clinical presentation of acute viral respiratory infection includes cough, dyspnea, fever, and pleuritic chest pain. Viral etiologies of lower respiratory infection are less likely to cause sputum production, and if present, tends to be watery or scant. In contrast, sputum production tends to be mucopurulent when due to bacterial pneumonia. Clinical signs of viral respiratory illness include fever, rales (crackles) on auscultation, hypoxemia, and tachycardia. These four signs together have a positive predictive value of 57.1%, with fever as the strongest clinically predictive sign of a viral respiratory infection versus that of bacterial etiology. Typically, patients with viral pneumonia also will present with a normal leukocyte count and bilateral pulmonary infiltrates on chest radiograph. Severe viral pneumonia can manifest as sepsis and respiratory distress requiring intensive care. In many moderate to severe cases of pneumonia, hypoxemia occurs from impaired alveolar gas exchange, often necessitating mechanical ventilation.

Several studies have documented SARS-CoV-2 infection in patients who never develop symptoms (asymptomatic) and in patients not yet symptomatic (pre-symptomatic). Since asymptomatic persons are not routinely tested, the prevalence of asymptomatic infection and detection of pre-symptomatic infection is not well understood. One study found that as many as 13% of RT-PCR-confirmed cases of SARS-CoV-2 infection in children were asymptomatic. Another study of skilled nursing facility residents infected with SARS-CoV-2 from a healthcare worker demonstrated that half were asymptomatic or pre-symptomatic at the time of contact tracing evaluation and testing. Patients may have abnormalities on chest imaging before the onset of symptoms. Some data suggest that pre-symptomatic infection tended to be detected in younger individuals and was less likely to be associated with viral pneumonia (https://www.cdc.gov/coronavirus/2019-ncov/hcp/clinical-guidance-management-patients.html).

Epidemiologic studies have documented SARS-CoV-2 transmission during the pre-symptomatic incubation period, and asymptomatic transmission has been suggested in other reports [28–30]. Virologic studies have also detected SARS-CoV-2 with RT-PCR low cycle thresholds, indicating larger quantities of viral RNA, and cultured viable virus among persons with asymptomatic and pre-symptomatic SARS-CoV-2 infection. The exact degree of SARS-CoV-2 viral RNA shedding that confers risk of transmission is not yet clear. Risk of transmission is thought to be greatest when patients are symptomatic since viral shedding is greatest at the time of symptom onset and declines over the course of several days to weeks. However, the proportion of SARS-CoV-2 transmission in the population due to asymptomatic or pre-symptomatic infection compared to symptomatic infection is unclear (https://www.uptodate.com/contents/coronavirus-disease-2019-covid-19-epidemiology-virology-and-prevention).

Biopsies in pneumonia are not routinely performed due to the lack of diagnostic, prognostic, and treatment value. However, since influenza has caused the most viral respiratory epidemics to date, a number of studies have examined infected patient's lung biopsy specimens. Biopsies obtained during influenza infection reveal a wide range of pathologies, including alveolar edema and exudate, interstitial inflammatory infiltration, and ulceration of bronchial mucosa to type II cell metaplasia. In autopsy specimens from H1N1 influenza patients, the respiratory tract exhibited tracheitis, bronchitis, diffuse hemorrhagic alveolar damage, and inflammatory infiltration of alveolar ducts and alveoli.

Since the COVID-19 caused by the novel coronavirus known as SARS-CoV-2 began its rapid spread in Wuhan, China, in November 2019, researchers have responded swiftly to help thwart the pandemic by quickly establishing studies to better understand the virus. SARS-CoV-2 is a novel beta-coronavirus that likely originated in bats. The virus uses a glycosylated spike protein to bind to and enter the human host cell predominantly via angiotensin-converting enzyme two receptors that are highly expressed in type 2 alveolar cells.

All testing for SARS-CoV-2 should be conducted in consultation with a healthcare provider. Specimens should be collected as soon as possible once a decision has been made to pursue testing, regardless of the time of symptom onset. For initial diagnostic testing for SARS-CoV-2, CDC recommends collecting and testing an upper respiratory specimen. The following are acceptable specimens:

- A nasopharyngeal (NP) specimen collected by a healthcare provider; or
- An oropharyngeal (OP) specimen collected by a healthcare provider; or
- A nasal mid-turbinate swab collected by a healthcare provider or by a supervised onsite self-collection (using a flocked tapered swab); or

- An anterior nares (nasal swab) specimen collected by a healthcare provider or by onsite or home self-collection (using a flocked or spun polyester swab); or
- Nasopharyngeal wash/aspirate or nasal wash/aspirate (NW) specimen collected by a healthcare provider.

Swabs should be placed immediately into a sterile transport tube containing 2–3 mL of either viral transport medium (VTM), Amies transport medium, or sterile saline, unless using a test designed to analyze a specimen directly (i.e., without placement in VTM), such as some point-of-care testsexternal icon.

The NW specimen and the non-bacteriostatic saline used to collect the specimen should be placed immediately into a sterile transport tube.

Testing lower respiratory tract specimens is also an option. For patients who develop a productive cough, sputum should be collected and tested for SARS-CoV-2. The induction of sputum is not recommended. When under certain clinical circumstances (e.g., those receiving invasive mechanical ventilation), a lower respiratory tract aspirate or bronchoalveolar lavage sample should be collected and tested as a lower respiratory tract specimen.

For providers collecting specimens or within 1.80 m or 6 ft. of patients suspected to be infected with SARS-CoV-2, maintain proper infection control and use recommended personal protective equipment (PPE), which includes an N95 or higher-level respirator (or facemask if a respirator is not available), eye protection, gloves, and a gown, when collecting specimens.

For providers who are handling specimens, but are not directly involved in collection (e.g., self-collection) and not working within 1.80 m or 6 ft. of the patient, follow Standard Precautions; gloves are recommended. Healthcare personnel are recommended to wear a form of source control (facemask or cloth face covering) at all times while in the healthcare facility (https://www.cdc.gov/coronavirus/2019-ncov/hcp/infection-control-recommendations.html).

PPE use can be minimized through patient self-collection while the healthcare provider maintains at least 6 ft. of separation.

5.13 Viral Pneumoniae Diagnosis: Upper Respiratory Sample Collection

Sterile swabs for upper respiratory specimen collection may be packaged in one of two ways:

- Individually wrapped (preferred when possible)
- Bulk packaged

Bulk-packaged swabs may be used for sample collection; however, care must be exercised to avoid SARS-CoV-2 contamination of any of the swabs in the bulk-packaged container.

- Before engaging with patients and while wearing a clean set of protective gloves, distribute individual swabs from the bulk container into individual disposable plastic bags

- If bulk-packaged swabs cannot be individually packaged:
  - Use only fresh, clean gloves to retrieve a single new swab from the bulk container.
  - Close the bulk swab container after each swab removal and leave it closed when not in use to avoid inadvertent contamination.
  - Store opened packages in a closed, airtight container to minimize contamination.
  - Keep all used swabs away from the bulk swab container to avoid contamination.
- As with all swabs, only grasp the swab by the distal end of the handle, using gloved hands only.
- When patients are self-collecting their swabs under clinical supervision:
  - Hand a swab to the patient only while wearing a clean set of protective gloves.
  - The patient can then self-swab and place the swab in transport media or sterile transport device and seal.
  - If the patient needs assistance, you can help the patient place the swab into transport media or a transport device and seal it.

5.13.1 Nasopharyngeal Swab/Oropharyngeal (Throat) Swab (Fig. 5.10)

NP swab: Insert minitip swab with a flexible shaft (wire or plastic) through the nostril parallel to the palate (not upwards) until resistance is encountered or the distance is equivalent to that from the ear to the nostril of the patient, indicating contact with the nasopharynx. Swab should reach depth equal to distance from nostrils to outer opening of the ear. Gently rub and roll the swab. Leave swab in place for several seconds to absorb secretions. Slowly remove swab while rotating it. Specimens can be collected from both sides using the same swab, but it is not necessary to collect specimens from both sides if the minitip is saturated with fluid from the first collection. If a deviated septum or blockage create difficulty in obtaining the specimen from one nostril, use the same swab to obtain the specimen from the other nostril.

OP swab: Insert swab into the posterior pharynx and tonsillar areas. Rub swab over both tonsillar pillars and posterior oropharynx and avoid touching the tongue, teeth, and gums.

5.13.2 Nasal Mid-Turbinate (NMT) Swab, Also Called Deep Nasal Swab

Use a flocked tapered swab. Tilt patient's head back 70°. While gently rotating the swab, insert swab less than 1 in. (about 2 cm) into nostril (until resistance is met at turbinates). Rotate the swab several times against nasal wall and repeat in other nostril using the same swab.

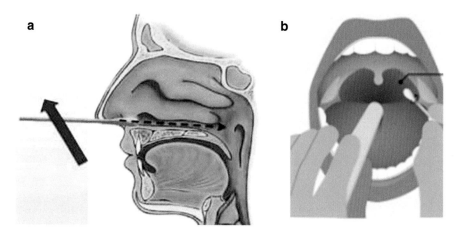

Fig. 5.10 (a) Procedure for taking material from the nasopharyngeal region, Nasopharyngeal swab. Photo donated by Dr. Di Lella Filippo of the ENT clinic of Parma. (b) Procedure for withdrawing material from the oropharyngeal region: oropharyngeal swab (throat). Photo donated by Dr. Di Lella Filippo of the ENT clinic of Parma

Fig. 5.11 Procedure for taking material from the anterior nostrils. Sample of anterior nostrils. Photo donated by Dr. Di Lella Filippo of the ENT clinic of Parma

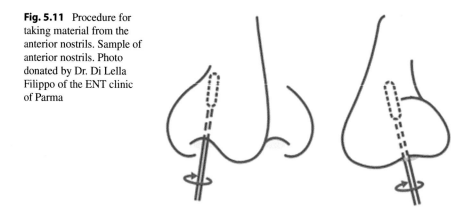

Anterior nares specimen (Fig. 5.11): Using a flocked or spun polyester swab, insert the swab at least 1 cm (0.5 in.) inside the nostril (naris) and firmly sample the nasal membrane by rotating the swab and leaving in place for 10–15 s. Sample both nostrils with same swab.

5.13.3 Nasopharyngeal Wash/Aspirate or Nasal Wash/Aspirate (Fig. 5.12)

Attach catheter to suction apparatus. Have the patient sit with head tilted slightly backward. Instill 1–1.5 mL of non-bacteriostatic saline (pH 7.0) into one nostril. Insert the tubing into the nostril parallel to the palate (not upwards). Catheter should reach depth equal to distance from nostrils to outer opening of ear. Begin gentle suction/aspiration and remove catheter while rotating it gently. Place specimen in a sterile viral transport media tube.

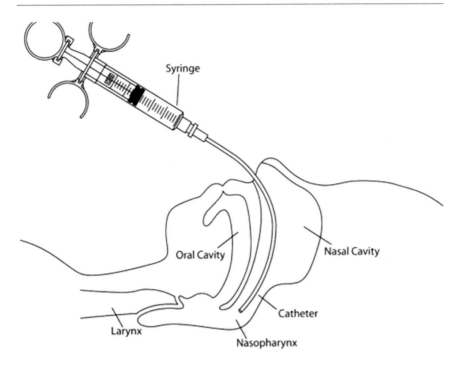

Fig. 5.12 Procedure for taking nasopharyngeal or nasal wash/aspiration material. Sample of Nasopharyngeal wash/aspiration or nasal wash/aspiration. Photo donated by Dr. Di Lella Filippo of the ENT clinic of Parma

Lower respiratory tract: *Bronchoalveolar lavage, tracheal aspirate, pleural fluid, lung biopsy.*

Collect 2–3 mL into a sterile, leak-proof, screw-cap sputum collection cup or sterile dry container.

Due to the increased technical skill and equipment needs, collection of specimens other than sputum from the lower respiratory tract may be limited to patients presenting with more severe disease, including people admitted to the hospital and/or fatal cases.

5.13.4 Sputum

Educate the patient about the difference between sputum and oral secretions (saliva). Have the patient rinse the mouth with water and then expectorate deep cough sputum directly into a sterile, leak-proof, screw-cap collection cup or sterile dry container.

5.13.5 Storage

Store specimens at 2–8 °C for up to 72 h after collection. If a delay in testing or shipping is expected, store specimens at −70 °C or below.

There are limited publications on the autopsy results of patients who have died from COVID-19. However, pathologic samples show hyaline membrane formation, interstitial mononuclear inflammatory infiltrates, and multinucleated giant cells. There are also high levels of pro-inflammatory cytokines, such as IL-2 and TNF-α. As with other causes of severe viral pneumonia, a "cytokine storm" occurs which also contributes to the high morbidity and mortality. Inflammatory infiltrate, edema, pneumocytic hyperplasia, fibrinous exudate and organization were found.

Despite the relevance of lung involvement in patients with COVID-19, few data regarding lung disease are available. In a clinical case of a deceased patient COVID-19 in China, histological findings in the lungs included desquamation of pneumocytes, diffuse alveolar damage, and edema. In addition, Tian and colleagues described the early stage lung disease COVID-19 in two patients with lung cancer; both patients showed signs of the widespread exudative phase alveolar damage. Fibrin thrombus in small arterial vessels (<1 mm in diameter) were observed in 87% of cases, approximately half of which had an involvement of over 25% of the lung tissue and high levels of D-dimers in the blood. These results could explain the severe hypoxemia that characterizes ARDS in vascular COVID-19. A patient's microthrombi are often identified in widespread areas of alveolar damage and are associated with diffuse endothelial damage. These features, although not pathognomonic, were frequent in the series, widespread in lung samples from the patients examined, and predominant distinctive vascular component. COVID-19 is complicated by coagulopathy and thrombosis. Furthermore, the D-dimer values of more than 1 μg/mL have been associated with fatal results in patients with COVID-19. For these reasons, the use of anticoagulants has been suggested to be potentially beneficial in patients with severe COVID-19, thanks also to their anti-inflammatory properties, although their effectiveness and safety have been carefully monitored. In an Italian study, they looked for virions in a subset of patients, and found virion-like particles present in the cytoplasm of pneumocytes and macrophages. The morphology of the observed particles (about 80 nm in diameter, wrapped, with pointed projections and an electron-lucent core with peripheral granules full of sectioned electrons nucleocapsid) and their intravacuolar cytoplasmic position are consistent with the reported ultrastructural coronavirus characteristics, including SARS-CoV2. Despite the low number of cases evaluated, these results suggest that the virus remains in the lung tissue for many days, albeit in small quantities, and it could trigger the mechanism leading to lung damage and it makes it progress. Further histological and molecular case series are being analyzed and extended to better define the cellular and tissue distribution of the virus and inflammatory responses into several organs. Although this report represents the largest European study of pulmonary autopsy results from COVID-19 cases based on the analysis of a large number of lung samples there is in it the limit of an absence of controls. All cases showed features of the exudative and proliferative phases of diffuse alveolar damage, which included capillary congestion (in all cases), pneumocyte necrosis (in all cases), hyaline membranes (in 33 cases), interstitial and intra-alveolar edema (in 37 cases), pneumocytic hyperplasia type 2 (in all cases), squamous metaplasia with atypia (in 21 cases), and thrombin-thrombin platelets (in 33 cases). The inflammatory infiltrate, observed in all cases, was largely composed of macrophages in the alveolar lumina (in 24 cases) and lymphocytes in the interstitium (in 31 cases). Electron microscopy revealed that the viral particles were mainly located in the pneumocytes. Interpretation: The predominant pattern of lung injury in patients with COVID-19 is diffuse alveolar damage, as described in patients with severe acute respiratory syndrome and middle respiratory syndrome infection with coronavirus. Hyaline membrane formation and atypical pneumocyte hyperplasia are frequent. Importantly, the presence of thrombin-platelet fibrin in small arterial vessels is consistent with coagulopathy, which appears to be common in patients with COVID-19 and should be a major goal of therapy [31].

References

1. Sprung J, Gajic O, Warner DO. Review article: age-related alterations in respiratory function-anaesthetic considerations. Can J Anaeth. 2006;53:1244–57.
2. Nagaratnam N, Nagaratnam K, Cheuk G. Diseases in the elderly—age-related changes and pathophysiology. Cham, Switzerland: Springer International Publishing; 2016.
3. Scheld WM, Mandell GI. Nosocomial pneumonia: pathogenesis and recent advances in diagnosis and therapy. Rev Infect Dis. 1991;13(Suppl 9):S743–51.
4. Emori TG, Banerjee SN, Culver DH, Gaynes RP, Horan TC, Edwards JR, et al. Nosocomial infections in the elderly patients in the United States. 1986–1990. Am J Med. 1991;91(S3B):289S–93S.
5. Schaaf B, Liebau C, Kurowski V, Droemann D, Dalhoff CK. Hospital acquired pneumonia with high-risk bacteria is associated with increased pulmonary matrix metalloproteinase activity. BMC Pulm Med. 2008;8:12.
6. Goldman-Cecil: Medicine 26th Ediction Elsevier 2020.
7. Ramirez JA, Wiemken TL, Peyrani P, et al. Adults hospitalized with pneumonia in the United States: incidence, epidemiology, and mortality. Clin Infect Dis. 2017;65:1806–12.
8. Torres A, Cillóniz C. Clinical management of bacterial pneumonia. Cham, Switzerland: Springer International Publishing; 2015. p. 1.
9. Berk SL. Bacterial pneumonia in the elderly: the observations of Sir William Osler in retrospect. J Am Geriatr Soc. 1984;32(9):683–5.
10. Henyg O, Keith S. Kaye Bacterial pneumoniae in older adult. Infect Dis Clin N Am. 2017;31:689–714.
11. https://www.medscape.com/answers/2500119-197502/what-are-the-symptoms-of-patients-with-coronavirus-disease-2019-covid-19.
12. CDC 02/06/2020: Interim Clinical Guidance for Management of Patients with Confirmed Coronavirus Disease COVID-19.
13. Gattinoni L, Chiumello D, Caironi P, et al. COVID-19 pneumonia: different respiratory treatments for different phenotypes? Intensive Care Med. 2020;46:1099–102. https://doi.org/10.1007/s00134-020-06033-2.
14. Ziehr DR, Alladina J, Petri CR, et al. Respiratory pathophysiology of mechanically ventilated patients with COVID-19: a cohort study. Am J Respir Crit Care Med. 2020; https://doi.org/10.1164/rccm.202004-1163LE.
15. Brown SM, Jones BE, Jephson AR, Dean NC. Validation of the Infectious Disease Society of America/American Thoracic Society 2007 guidelines for severe community-acquired pneumonia. Crit Care Med. 2009;37(12):3010–6.
16. Fang WF, Yang KY, Wu CL, Yu CJ, Chen CW, Tu CY, et al. Application and comparison of scoring indices to predict outcomes in patients with healthcare-associated pneumonia. Crit Care. 2011;15(1):R32.
17. Fine MJ, Auble TE, Yealy DM, Hanusa BH, Weissfeld LA, Singer DE, et al. A prediction rule to identify low-risk patients with community-acquired pneumonia. N Engl J Med. 1997;336(4):243–50.

18. Cillóniz C, Ewig S, Polverino E, Marcos MA, Esquinas C, Gabarrús A, et al. Microbial aetiology of community-acquired pneumonia and its relation to severity. Thorax. 2011;66(4):340–6.
19. Song J-H, et al. Treatment guidelines for community-acquired pneumonia in Korea: an evidence-based approach to appropriate antimicrobial therapy. Infect Chemother. 2009;41(3):133–53. https://doi.org/10.3947/ic.2009.41.3.133.
20. Sligl WI, Majumdar SR, Marrie TJ. Triaging severe pneumonia: what is the "score" on prediction rules? Crit Care Med. 2009;37(12):3166–8.
21. Liang W, Liang H, Ou L, et al. Development and validation of a clinical risk score to predict the occurrence of critical illness in hospitalized patients with COVID-19. JAMA Intern Med. 2020;2020:e202033. https://doi.org/10.1001/jamainternmed.2020.2033.
22. Wootton D, Feldman C. The diagnosis of pneumonia requires a chest radiograph (X-ray)—yes, no or sometimes? Pneumonia. 2014;5:1–7. https://doi.org/10.15172/pneu.2014.5/464.
23. Henig O, Kaye KS. Bacterial pneumonia in older adults. Infect Dis Clin N Am. 2017;31(4):689–713. https://doi.org/10.1016/j.idc.2017.07.015.
24. Chavez MA, Shams N, Ellington LE, et al. Lung ultrasound for the diagnosis of pneumonia in adults: a systematic review and meta-analysis. Respir Res. 2014;15:50.
25. Seo H, Cha S-I, Shin K-M, Lim J-K, Yoo S-S, Lee S-Y, Lee J, Kim C-H, Park J-Y. Community-acquired pneumonia with negative chest radiography findings: clinical and radiological features. Respiration. 2019;97:508–17. https://doi.org/10.1159/000495068.
26. Ticinesi A, Lauretani F, Nouvenne A, et al. Lung ultrasound and chest X-ray for detecting pneumonia in an acute geriatric ward. Medicine. 2016;95(27):e4153.
27. Gadsby NJ, Russell CD, McHugh MP, et al. Comprehensive molecular testing for respiratory pathogens in community-acquired pneumonia. Clin Infect Dis. 2016;62:817–23.
28. Jain S, Self WH, Wunderink RG, et al. Community-acquired pneumonia requiring hospitalization among U.S. adults. N Engl J Med. 2015;373:415–27.
29. Oyarzun GM. Pulmonary function in aging. Rev Med Chil. 2009;137:411–8; (abstract)
30. Fry AM, Shay DK, Holman RC, et al. Trends in hospitalizations for pneumonia among persons aged 65 years or older in the United States, 1988-2002. JAMA. 2005;294(21):2712–9.
31. Carsana L, Sonzogni A, Nasr A, Rossi RS, Pellegrinelli A, Zerbi P, Rech R, Colombo R, Antinori S, Corbellino M, Galli M, Catena E, Tosoni A, Gianatti A, Nebuloni M. Pulmonary post-mortem findings in a series of COVID-19 cases from northern Italy: a two-centre descriptive study. Lancet Infect Dis. 2020; https://doi.org/10.1016/S1473-3099(20)30434-5.

The Diagnosis of COVID ARF in Elderly: The Radiological Findings in Elderly

6

Tullio Valente and Federica Romano

Key Points
- Older patients are at particular risk of having COVID-19 severe infection, and have a higher mortality.
- In addition to age, male gender, and presence of comorbidities, specific radiological findings are important prognostic factors.
- Imaging features help in evaluation of the severity and extent of the disease.

6.1 Introduction

In December 2019, a highly infectious disease emerged in the city of Wuhan in Hubei province, China, which was later proven to have been caused by a novel coronavirus (2019-nCoV or SARS-CoV-2) [1]. The WHO christened the disease as COVID-19 and declared it as a pandemic on March 11, 2020. In the following weeks, the disease has swept rapidly across most of the countries of the world causing a global health emergency. Viral polymerase chain reaction (PCR) and serology are the mainstays of testing, but a positive diagnosis may be increasingly supported by imaging findings. This review is retrospectively performed to identify the key imaging manifestations, distribution, temporal evolution, and complications of the lesions in the elderly (>65 years) patients with COVID-19 pneumonia.

T. Valente (✉) · F. Romano
Department of Radiology, Azienda Ospedali dei Colli, Monaldi Hospital, Naples, Italy

N. Vargas, A. M. Esquinas (eds.), *Covid-19 Airway Management and Ventilation Strategy for Critically Ill Older Patients*, https://doi.org/10.1007/978-3-030-55621-1_6

67

6.2   Radiology of the Normal Aging Lung and COVID-19 Disease

The world aging population is continuously rising and Italy is the second country following Japan with the largest concentration of persons living over the age of 65 years.

Lung function declines in the elderly, and lung aging is accompanied by functional and morphologic-structural changes. Chest X-ray (CXR) studies have found increased peripheral lung markings with increasing age [2]. Thin-section high-resolution computed tomography of the chest (HRCT) provides greater anatomic detail and allows increased sensitivity and specificity in comparison to CXR in a range of pulmonary conditions, including lung physiological aging process structural aspects [3–6]. HRCT findings usually seen in asymptomatic older individuals are shown in Table 6.1. One large study observed the death rate to be more than double in the over 65s (hazard ratio 2.43, 95% confidence interval 1.66–3.56) [7] .

6.3   Chest Imaging in Elderly COVID-19 Patients

The novel coronavirus has a specific tropism for the low respiratory airways and the main complication of the disease is pneumonia. Thoracic imaging plays a pivotal role in diagnosis, temporal evolution, complications, monitoring of therapeutic efficacy, and elderly COVID-19 patients discharge assessment.

- Chest X-Ray *(CXR).*

Portable CXR is typically the first-line imaging modality, helpful for critically ill patients who are immobile. Daily routine portable CXR are recommended for critically ill ICU patients. In non-severe clinical disease, up to 18% of patients have a normal initial CXR or CT, but only 3% in severe disease [8]. Of elderly patients with COVID-19 who required hospitalization, 80% had radiographic abnormalities sometime during hospitalization.

The most frequent CXR signs are patchy or diffuse asymmetric, ill-defined margins, airspace opacities, whether described as consolidation or, less commonly, as GGO areas which peaked at 10–12 days from symptom onset. The distribution is

Table 6.1 Prevalence of thin-section CT findings in asymptomatic older (>65 years) non-smokers and ex-smokers individuals (percentages in parentheses)

• Reticular pattern (mild interstitial fibrosis) and focal parenchymal abnormalities like septal thickening (60%)
• Parenchymal bands (50%)
• Bronchial dilation and wall thickening (55–60%)
• Cysts (25%)
• Centrilobular emphysema (5%)
• Air-trapping (15%)

most often bilateral, peripheral, and lower zone predominant [9, 10]. CXR findings are not organism specific and can overlap with other causes of viral or atypical pneumonia.

The extent of pulmonary abnormalities may be unilateral or multi-lobar (more than two lobes), and bilateral involvement; it maybe semiquantitatively graded as the percentage of each zone involved and an average calculated for each radiologic study [11] (Fig. 6.1). In contrast to parenchymal abnormalities, pleural effusion is rare (3%).

- Lung Ultrasound (LUS).

Lung US is a surface imaging technique greatly developed in the last decades and strongly recommended for acute respiratory failure [12]. This technique is used in emergency room setting and intensive care unit (ICU) patients in supine (ventral thorax) and, depending on the clinic, in a sitting position (dorsal thorax). Bedside LUS has a major utility for the management of COVID-19 pneumonia due to its safety, repeatability, low cost, and point of care use. Moreover, ultrasonic pocket device has advantages over CT and CXR in disinfection and smaller area of contact with patients. According to the Bedside Lung Ultrasound in Emergency-PLUS protocol, LUS 12-area examination method is adopted, in which a lung is divided by the anterior axillary and posterior axillary lines into three areas: anterior, lateral, and posterior (each lung is divided into six areas) [13].

The LUS main findings in COVID-19 pneumonia include all those which are well known in acute respiratory distress syndrome (ARDS). Greater specificity to LUS signs is given by the patchy distribution (multiform clusters of findings and sharply alternated to spared normal areas) and the current epidemiological milieu, clinically characterized by flulike symptoms. The diagnosis of lung pathologies relies on the artifacts of subpleural peri-pulmonary lesions:

- Thickening of the pleural line with pleural line irregularity; the serosa can be unsmooth, discontinuous, and fragmented, as is commonly observed in ARDS
- B-lines are visualized as a storm of clusters of B-lines (B-pattern), both in separate and coalescent fused forms, sometimes giving the appearance of a shining white lung. These lines correspond to the early appearance of "ground glass" areas detected in CT, and can often arise from one point of the thickened pleural line and from small peripheral consolidations (Fig. 6.2).

In early phase of the disease, often B-lines move rapidly with sliding, appear and disappear (waterfall or light beam sign), at times creating an "on–off" effect in the context of an often normal A-lines lung pattern visible on the background [14, 15]. These artifacts occur because of the abnormal sound wave reflection caused by changes in the ratio of air and water contents in alveoli (reduced air content) and thickened/edematous interstitial tissues due to COVID-19 pneumonia predominant posterior subpleural lesions. B-lines, while representing typical signs of the disease, can be found in other interstitial diseases of various etiologies.

- In summary, bilateral, patchy distribution of multiple cluster areas with the waterfall/light beam sign, alternating with areas with multiple separated and coalescent B-lines and well-demarcated separation from large "spared" areas.

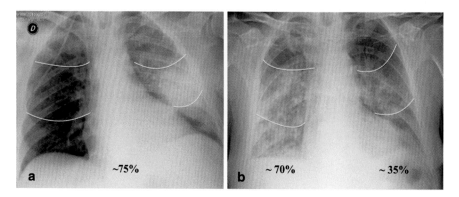

Fig. 6.1 CXR semiquantitative pneumonia lung involvement evaluation. Each lung can be divided into an upper, middle, and lower zone (each comprising 1/3 of the cranial-caudal lung extension on AP radiography and a zonal involvement can be assigned. (**a**) About a 75% of the left lung volume involvement is seen. (**b**) On the right hemithorax about a 70% of the left lung volume involvement is seen; on the left hemithorax about a 35% of the left lung is seen

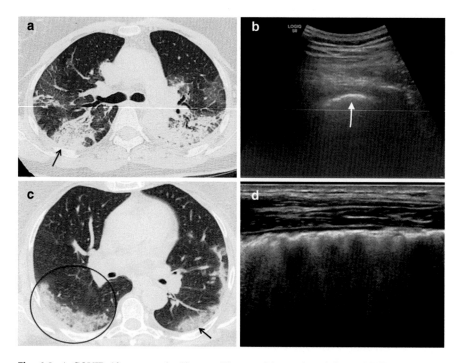

Fig. 6.2 A COVID-19 pneumonia 68-year-old man with cough and fever (38.2°). (**a**) HRCT image shows ground-glass opacity and air bronchogram sign under the pleura in the posterior lower field of the right lung (arrow). (**b**) The convex array probe shows **b**-lines and waterfall sign in the right posterior upper area (arrow), and the unsmooth and thickened pleural line. (**c**) A COVID-19 pneumonia 73-year-old man with cough and fever (38.5°). HRCT image shows bilateral GGO areas, cloudy shadows under the pleura in the posterior lower lobes, air bronchogram sign, and air bronchiologram sign (red circle on the right lung and arrow on the left lung). (**d**) The 9–15 MHz high-frequency linear array probe clearly shows the thickened and rough irregular pleural line in the right lower lobe GGO area and thin with diffused **b**-lines

- Multifocal mainly posterior subpleural small consolidations in different patterns, including consolidations up to non-translobar and translobar with occasional dynamic air bronchograms.
- Large tissue-like consolidation without bronchograms (obstructive atelectasis).
- Spared areas are present bilaterally, mixed with pathological areas.
- Sliding is usually preserved in all but severe cases.
- Large (simple or complex) pleural effusions are uncommon in COVID-19 disease.

LUS can be used for rapid assessment of COVID-19 pneumonia typical manifestations, to track the evolution of disease during follow-up and to monitor lung recruitment maneuvers. LUS has advantages over bedside CXR, but it cannot fully replace CT.

- Thin-Slice CT/HRCT.

Thin-section or high-resolution CT (HRCT) is of outstanding importance as it is the main tool for new coronavirus pneumonia baseline early diagnosis, evaluation of disease severity, temporal evolution, and therapeutic response. CT findings are used mainly according to Fleischner Society glossary of terms for thoracic imaging (Table 6.2) [16].

CT has been used as an important complement to RT-PCR (real-time polymerase chain reaction) for diagnosing COVID-19 pneumonia in the current epidemic context [17]. Indeed, when the viral load is insufficient, RT-PCR can be falsely negative while chest CT shows suggestive abnormalities [18]. However, CT sensitivity is also dependent on the time course of symptoms.

According to the literature [19–28] four temporal evolution CT stages on COVID-19 elderly patients have been described, such as their characteristic findings:

(a) *Early/initial stage* (0–4 days): normal CT (about 30% within 2 days of symptom onset) or a pattern characterized by:
    - Ground-glass opacities (GGO), whether isolated or coexisting with minor consolidations, lungs (in 57% of elderly patients) (Fig. 6.3).
    - Main ancillary thoracic CT findings in this stage of the disease were pulmonary vascular enlargement (84%), intralobular septal thickening (50%), adjacent pleural thickening (40%), air bronchograms (40%), subpleural lines (25%), and crazy-paving pattern (15%) (Fig. 6.4).
    - The incidence of consolidation, linear opacities, and crazy-paving pattern in severe/critical patients is significantly higher than that observed in non-severe patients.
(b) *Progressive stage* (5–8 days):
    - Increased GGO and crazy-paving appearance; sometimes reverse halo sign may be associated.
    - Younger people tend to have more GGOs, while older or sicker people tend to have more extensive involvement with consolidations.

Table 6.2 Glossary of terms for thoracic imaging used in COVID-19 pneumonia (HR) CT reports

CT finding	Definition
Air bronchogram	A pattern of air-filled (low-attenuation) bronchi on a background of opaque (high-attenuation)
Airspace	The gas-containing part of the lung, including the respiratory bronchioles but excluding purely conducting airways
Airway changes	Include bronchiectasis and bronchial wall thickening
Consolidation	An exudate or other product of disease that replaces alveolar air in the airspaces, rendering the lung solid and obscuring bronchovascular margins
Crazy-paving pattern	Thickened interlobular septa and intralobular lines superimposed on a background of ground-glass opacity
Fibrosis	Fibrous stripes forming during the healing of pulmonary chronic inflammation or proliferative disease, with gradual replacement of cellular components by scar tissues
Ground-glass opacity (GGO)	Hazy increased opacity of lung, with preservation of bronchial and vascular margins
Diffuse alveolar damage (DAD)	The acute phase is characterized by edema and hyaline membrane formation. The later phase is characterized by airspace and/or interstitial organization
Interlobular septum	A sheetlike structure 10–20-mm long that form the borders of secondary lobule
Organizing pneumonia (OP) pattern	Typically subpleural and basal, sometimes bronchocentric, GGO and consolidation areas by loose plugs of connective tissue in the airspaces and distal airways
Parenchymal band or subpleural line	A curvilinear line opacity, usually 1–3 mm thick and up to 5 cm long that usually extends to the visceral pleura
Reticular pattern	A collection of innumerable small linear opacities that, by summation, produce an appearance resembling a net
Reverse halo sign	A GGO area surrounded by peripheral annular consolidation
Secondary pulmonary lobule	The smallest unit of lung surrounded by connective tissue septa
Vascular enlargement	The dilatation of pulmonary vessels around and within the hyperdense lung lesions

- The proportion of multiple lobe involvement in the elderly group is higher than that in the young and middle-aged group.
(c) *Peak stage* (9–13 days):
- Progression of GGOs into consolidation and a mixed pattern, sometimes associated with superimposed intralobular reticulation resulting in a crazy-paving pattern.
- The lesions showed mild to moderate progression along the initial 2 weeks from symptom onset.
- A thin hypoattenuating line in between the visceral pleura and the high-density lesion or subpleural sparing is seen in 55% of the patients.

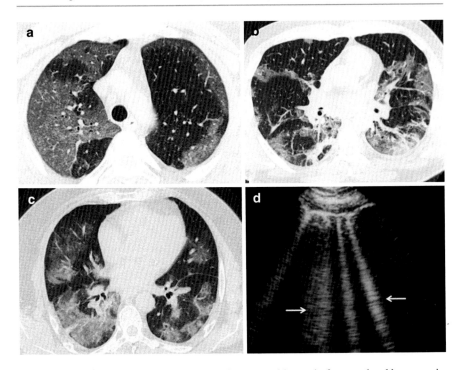

Fig. 6.3 A COVID-19 pneumonia 69-year-old woman with cough, fever, and sudden anosmia. (**a–c**) Basilar HRCT axial image 2 days after symptoms onset (early stage) shows large patchy subpleural bilateral GGO areas. CT involvement is 14/24. (**d**) The convex array probe reveals fixed coalescent discontinuous **b**-lines (waterfall sign) in the left posterior lower lobe (arrows)

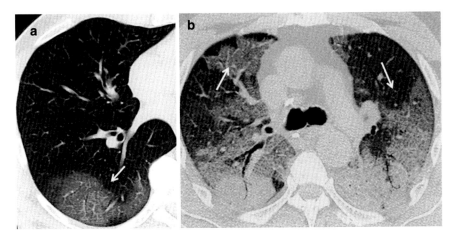

Fig. 6.4 Ancillary lung main CT findings in early stage COVID-19 pneumonia. (**a**) HRCT close-view image shows a «bronchus» sign and «vascular enlargement» sign in a subpleural posterior GGO area of right lower lobe in a 68-year-old man (arrow). (**b**) HRCT image shows bilateral crazy-paving pattern in another elderly patient (arrows)

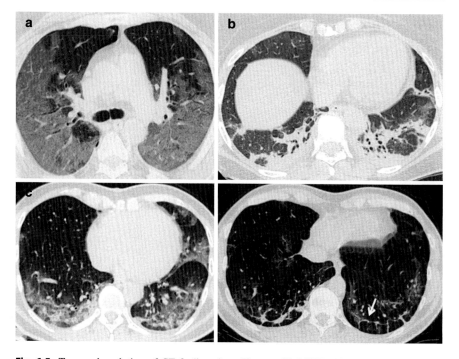

Fig. 6.5 Temporal evolution of CT findings in a 68-year-old COVID-19 pneumonia man with fever (38.5 °C) and acute respiratory failure; the patient was tachypneic (30 bpm), with lymphopenia and low oxygen saturation (SpO$_2$ 85%, PAFI < 250), required mechanical ventilation, and was admitted to intensive care unit. (**a**) Baseline (on admission, 1st day from symptoms onset) HRCT image shows extensive bilateral GGO areas involving both lungs consistent with severe pneumonia. CT involvement is 20/24. (**b**) Follow-up (8th day from symptoms onset) HRCT image shows a posterior mixed pattern (GGO and consolidation areas) in both lower lobes. CT involvement is 16/24. (**c**) Follow-up (16th day from symptoms onset) HRCT image shows bilateral subpleural OP-like curvilinear consolidative parenchymal bands and mild GGO areas. CT involvement is 10/24. (**d**) Follow-up (42nd day from symptoms onset) HRCT image shows only bibasilar curvilinear fibrotic stripes (arrows). CT involvement is 4/24. The patient was discharged on the 44th day in good health

(d) *Absorption stage* (>14 days):
- With an improvement in the disease course, curvilinear subpleural enlarged fibrotic OP-like areas/stripes and architectural distortion appear (Fig. 6.5).
- The abnormalities resolve at 1 month and beyond or linear streaks of fibrosis remain.
- A total of 80% of the patients had residual lesions at the time of discharge, of which a majority are GGO and residual linear opacities.

According to Zhao W et al., we divide each lung into three zones: upper (above the carina), middle (below the carina up to the inferior pulmonary vein), and lower (below the inferior pulmonary vein) zones [29].

A semiquantitative CT severity score (CT-SS) is assigned for each lung zone: score 0, 0% involvement; score 1, less than 25% involvement; score 2, 25% to less than 50% involvement; score 3, 50% to less than 75% involvement; and score 4, 75% or greater involvement. There are 6 lung zones per patient; the maximal score is 4 times 6 zones resulting in a score of 24 [29]. The frequency of consolidations as well as the median CT-SS score have been both higher in the group of elderly patients who died at the hospital, as compared to patients who could be discharged. Critical cases may show further expanded consolidation, with the whole lung density showing increased opacity, sometimes known as a "white lung." In addition to the extension of the consolidations and the CT-SS score, other predictive factors for mortality include older age and higher comorbidity rate (e.g., the "frail elderly" individuals). ICU patients tend to be older and with more comorbidities.

– Cavitation (0.1%), pleural effusions (5%), mediastinal lymphadenopathy (5.0%), pericardial effusions (3.6%), and reversed halo sign (2.5) are less common manifestations of COVID-19. Centrilobular nodules, mucoid impactions and unilateral segmental or lobar consolidations suggest a bacterial origin of pneumonia, or superinfection.

6.4   Imaging of COVID-19 Pneumonia Complications

The cornerstone of therapy for pneumonia is respiratory support with both noninvasive (NIV) or invasive (IV) ventilation, or extracorporeal membrane oxygenation (ECMO). In patients with a marked elevation of d-dimers and clinical worsening not explained by an extension of lung opacities on CT, pulmonary embolism should be suspected and a contrast-enhanced CT examination should be performed, always taking into consideration the clinical severity and the renal function. These critically ill patients should be treated accordingly and monitored by cardiac and venous ultrasound to diagnose deep venous thrombosis and cardiac signs of acute pulmonary embolism.

COVID-19 patients with severe infection can develop a pro-inflammatory cytokine release syndrome, which can lead to rapid deterioration and fatal acute respiratory distress syndrome (ARDS). This is reported to occur in between 15% and 23% of cases [30, 31]. ARDS pattern represents a "final common pathway" of several lung injury, and diffuse alveolar damage (DAD) is regarded as its key pathological finding. Injury to the alveolar epithelial cells is the main cause of COVID-19-related ARDS, and endothelial cells seem to be less damaged with therefore less exudation. The onset time of COVID-19-related ARDS is 8–12 days. ARDS is the most common indication for transferring patients with COVID-19 infection to the ICU and the major cause of ICU death in these patients [32]. ARDS CT findings are well known [33].

6.5   Conclusion

In this epidemic situation, imaging (particularly CT) undoubtedly plays an important role, for early identification of COVID-19 pneumonia. Typical in elderly patients CT features include peripheral GGOs with multifocal distribution, and a progressive evolution towards organizing pneumonia patterns. LUS and CT may be used for prognosis purposes, with poorer outcome for patients having important disease extent and more consolidative forms and also to early detect complications in patients who require further mechanical ventilation.

Acknowledgments The authors declare no conflict of interest.

References

1. Zhu N, Zhang D, Wang WJ, et al. A novel coronavirus from patients with pneumonia in China, 2019. N Engl J Med. 2020;382:727–33. https://doi.org/10.1056/NEJMoa2001017.
2. Ensor RE, Fleg JL, Kim YC, de Leon EF, Goldman SM. Longitudinal chest x-ray changes in normal men. J Gerontol. 1983;38:307–14.
3. Copley SJ, Wells AU, Hawtin KE, Gibson DJ, Hodson JM, Jacques AET, Hansell DM. Lung morphology in the elderly: comparative CT study of subjects over 75 years old versus those under 55 years old. Radiology. 2009;251:566–73. https://doi.org/10.1148/radiol.2512081242.
4. Schröder TH, Storbeck B, Rabe KF, Weber C. The aging lung: clinical and imaging findings and the fringe of physiological state. RöFo. 2015;187:430–9. https://doi.org/10.1055/s-0034-1399227.
5. Winter DH, Manzini M, Salge JM, Busse A, Jaluul O, Filho WJ, Mathias W, Terra-Filho M. Aging of the lungs in asymptomatic lifelong nonsmokers: findings on HRCT. Lung. 2015;193:283–90. https://doi.org/10.1007/s00408-015-9700-3.
6. Copley SJ. Morphology of the aging lung on computed tomography. J Thorac Imaging. 2016;31:140–50. https://doi.org/10.1097/RTI.0000000000000211.
7. Cheng Y, Luo R, Wang K, et al. Kidney disease is associated with in-hospital death of patients with COVID-19. Kidney Int. 2020;97(5):829–38.
8. Guan WJ, Ni ZY, Hu Y, et al. Clinical characteristics of coronavirus disease 2019 in China. N Engl J Med. 2020;382:1708–20. https://doi.org/10.1056/NEJMoa2002032.
9. Wong HYF, Lam HYS, Fong AH, Leung ST, Chin TW, Lo CSY, Lui MM, Lee JCY, Chiu KW, Chung T, Lee EYP, Wan EYF, Hung FNI, Lam TPW, Kuo M, Ng MY. Frequency and distribution of chest radiographic findings in COVID-19 positive patients. Radiology. 2019;2:201160. https://doi.org/10.1148/radiol.2020201160.
10. Rodrigues JCL, Hareb SS, Edeyc A, Devarajd A, Jacobe J, Johnstoneg A, McStayh R, Nairi A, Robinson G. An update on COVID-19 for the radiologist—a British society of thoracic imaging statement. Clin Radiol. 2020;75:323–5. https://doi.org/10.1016/j.crad.2020.03.003.
11. Valente T, Lassandro F, Marino M, Squillante F, Aliperta M, Muto R. H1N1 pneumonia: our experience in 50 patients with a severe clinical course of novel swine-origin influenza a (H1N1) virus (S-OIV). Radiol Med. 2012;117:165–84. https://doi.org/10.1007/s11547-011-0734-1.
12. Mongodi S, Pozzi M, Orlando A, et al. Lung ultrasound for daily monitoring of ARDS patients on extracorporeal membrane oxygenation: preliminary experience. Intensive Care Med. 2018;44:123–4. https://doi.org/10.1007/s00134-017-4941-7.
13. Patel CJ, Bhatt HB, Parikh SN, Jhaveri BN, Puranik JH. Bedside lung ultrasound in emergency protocol as a diagnostic tool in patients of acute respiratory distress presenting to emergency department. J Emerg Trauma Shock. 2018;11(2):125–9. https://doi.org/10.4103/JETS.JETS_21_17.
14. Huang Y, Wang S, Liu Y, et al. A preliminary study on the ultrasonic manifestations of peripulmonary lesions of non-critical novel coronavirus pneumonia (COVID-19). SSRN. 2020; https://doi.org/10.2139/ssrn.3544750.
15. Volpicelli G, Gargani L. Sonographic signs and patterns of COVID-19 pneumonia. Ultrasound J. 2020;12:22. https://doi.org/10.1186/s13089-020-00171-w.
16. Hansell DM, Bankier AA, MacMahon H, McLoud TC, Müller NL, Remy J. Fleischner society: glossary of terms for thoracic imaging. Radiology. 2008;246:697–722. https://doi.org/10.1148/radiol.2462070712.

17. Fang Y, Zhang H, Xie J, Lin M, Ying L, Pang P, et al. Sensitivity of chest CT for COVID-19: comparison to RT-PCR. Radiology. 2020;2:200432. https://doi.org/10.1148/radiol.20202004.32.
18. Ai T, Yang Z, Hou H, Zhan C, Chen C, Lv W, et al. Correlation of chest CT and RT-PCR testing in coronavirus disease 2019 (COVID-19) in China: a report of 1014 cases. Radiology. 2020; https://doi.org/10.1148/radiol.2020200642.
19. Pan F, Ye T, Sun P, Gui S, Liang B, Li L, et al. Time course of lung changes on chest CT during recovery from 2019 novel coronavirus (COVID-19) Pneumonia. Radiology. 2020; https://doi.org/10.1148/radiol.2020200370.
20. Song F, Shi N, Shan F, Zhang Z, et al. Emerging 2019 novel coronavirus (2019-nCoV) pneumonia. Radiology. 2020;295(1):210–7.
21. Zhu T, Wang Y, Zhou S, Zhang N, Xia L. A comparative study of chest computed tomography features in young and older adults with corona virus disease (COVID-19). J Thorac Imaging. 2020;35:W97. https://doi.org/10.1097/RTI.0000000000000513.
22. Huang C, Wang Y, Li X, et al. Clinical features of patients infected with 2019 novel coronavirus in Wuhan, China. Lancet. 2020;395(10223):497–506.
23. Chung M, Bernheim A, Mei X, et al. CT imaging features of 2019 novel coronavirus (2019-nCoV). Radiology. 2020;295(1):202–7.
24. Shi H, Han X, Jiang N, et al. Radiological findings from 81 patients with COVID-19 pneumonia in Wuhan, China: a descriptive study. Lancet Infect Dis. 2020;20:425–34. https://doi.org/10.1016/S1473-3099(20)30086-4.
25. Liu KC, Xu P, Lv W-F, et al. CT manifestations of coronavirus disease-2019: a retrospective analysis of 73 cases by disease severity. Eur J Radiol. 2020;126:108941. https://doi.org/10.1016/j.ejrad.2020.108941.
26. Wang K, Kang S, Tian R, Zhang X, Zhang X, Wang Y. Imaging manifestations and diagnostic value of chest CT of coronavirus disease 2019 (COVID-19) in the Xiaogan area. Clin Radiol. 2020;75:341–7. https://doi.org/10.1016/j.crad.2020.03.004.
27. Guan CS, Lv ZB, Yan S, et al. Imaging features of coronavirus disease 2019 (COVID-19): evaluation on thin-section CT. Acad Radiol. 2020;27:609–13. https://doi.org/10.1016/j.acra.2020.03.002.
28. Ojha V, Mani A, Pandey NN, Kumar SS, Kumar S. CT in coronavirus disease 2019 (COVID-19): a systematic review of chest CT findings in 4410 adult patients. Eur Radiol. 2020; https://doi.org/10.1007/s00330-020-06975-7.
29. Zhao W, Zhong Z, Xie X, et al. Relation between chest CT findings and clinical conditions of coronavirus disease (COVID-19) pneumonia: a multicenter study. Am J Roentgenol. 2020;214:1072–7. https://doi.org/10.2214/AJR.20.22976.
30. Sun P, Qie S, Liu Z, Ren J, Jianing XJ. Clinical characteristics of 50466 patients with 2019-nCoV infection. medRxiv 2020;2020.02.18.20024539.
31. Qian K, Deng Y, Tai Y, Peng J, Peng H, Jiang L. Clinical characteristics of 2019 novel infected coronavirus pneumonia: a systemic review and meta-analysis. medRxiv 2020; 2020.02.14.20021535.
32. Salehi S, Abedi A, Balakrishnan S, Gholamrezanezhad A. Coronavirus disease 2019 (COVID-19): a systematic review of imaging findings in 919 patients. Am J Roentgenol. 2020;215:87–93. https://doi.org/10.2214/AJR.20.23034.
33. Zompatori M, Ciccarese F, Fasano L. Overview of current lung imaging in acute respiratory distress syndrome. Eur Respir Rev. 2014;23:519–30. https://doi.org/10.1183/09059180.00001314.

Part III

The Screening and the Access to ICU

The Screening and the Access to ICU

7

Maria Vargas, Rosario Sara, Pasquale Buonanno,
and Giuseppe Servillo

7.1 The Recommendations of the Intensive Caring Scientific Societies

A novel coronavirus was identified in late 2019 as the cause of a cluster of pneumonia cases in Wuhan, China. It has since rapidly spread resulting in a pandemic. The World Health Organization designated the disease term COVID-19 (Coronavirus Disease 2019). The virus that causes COVID-19 is designated severe acute respiratory syndrome coronavirus 2 (SARS-CoV-2). The major morbidity and mortality from COVID-19 is largely due to acute viral pneumonitis that evolves to acute respiratory distress syndrome (ARDS).

In some states of the world the epidemic has spread widely and heterogeneously for structural and geographical reasons.

In Germany, the outbreaks have been practically homogeneous in the various Landers. This, together with an adequate planning of the number of ICU beds (6/1000 inhabitants), has allowed the national system to respond adequately in quantitative terms.

In the USA and Italy, the spread of the virus has been very irregular. The state of New York and the Lombardy region have been involved in most part while other regions of the same states have had significantly less outbreaks. These concentrations of cases caused a dramatic collapse of the local health system, which, being unable to ensure adequate intensive care for the whole population, had to make transfers or tragic choices.

Manca D, from Lombardy, on 18 March affirmed that "There are no stationary days or decrease days during the Covid-19 emergency. The medical choices to intubate patients could have changed during the studied period, according to the

M. Vargas (✉) · R. Sara · P. Buonanno · G. Servillo
Department of Neurosciences, Reproductive Sciences and Odontostomatology,
University of Naples Federico II, Naples, Italy

© The Editor(s) (if applicable) and The Author(s), under exclusive license to
Springer Nature Switzerland AG 2020
N. Vargas, A. M. Esquinas (eds.), *Covid-19 Airway Management and Ventilation Strategy for Critically Ill Older Patients*, https://doi.org/10.1007/978-3-030-55621-1_7

hospital organization, to the availability of resources, and to recommendations, leading to an underestimation of the true necessity of NICUC (Covid ICU beds)." [1].

The increased knowledge of the virus and related pathology has led the Intensive Caring Scientific Societies to draw up new guidelines on patient access to ICU.

7.1.1 The Usual Screening and the Access to ICU

The decision to admit patients to intensive care or discharge them to a hospital ward (or even directly back home) is a daily task for intensivists, a life-changing event for patients and families, and in aggregate a major strategic issue for health care systems worldwide [2].

Indications for ICU admission should consider:

- Critical state in progress due to insufficiency of one or more vital functions (intensive treatment).
- High risk of developing a critical state due to the occurrence of serious and foreseeable complications (intensive monitoring).

Patients who need intensive treatment for an acute critical state have priority over patients who require intensive monitoring as well as critically ill patients with a worse prognosis [2].

Therefore, the necessary conditions for an ICU admission are severity, reversibility, evaluation of premorbid conditions, and, where possible, consent [3, 4].

With regard to gravity, all cases of insufficiency of vital functions (current or potential) that can lead to short-term death are included: respiratory arrest requiring mechanical ventilation; invasive monitoring and infusion of vasoactive drugs necessary to support cardiovascular function; invasive monitoring and deep sedation to preserve the nervous system; hemofiltration for kidney function; correction of toxic states by intake of substances; postoperative care of patients who require hemodynamic monitoring and/or ventilatory support; acute states from endocrine pathologies (ketoacidosis, acute adrenal insufficiency, etc.); septic shock, polytraumatized, burned and more that need intensive care.

Clinical signs that fall within the ICU admission criteria are:

- Heart rate <40 or >150 bpm; systolic blood pressure (SAP) <80 mmHg; mean blood pressure (MAP) <60 mmHg; diastolic blood pressure (DAP) >120 mmHg; respiratory rate (RR) >35 acts/min. General parameters show hemodynamic instability and must be analyzed on a case-by-case.

A lot of laboratory data can help us to select the patient who needs intensive care:
- Serum sodium <110 mEq/L or >170 mEq/L; serum potassium <2.0 mEq/L or >7.0 mEq/L; $PaO_2 < 50$ mmHg; pH < 7.1 or >7.7; blood glucose >800 mg/dL; calcemia >15 mg/dL; toxic levels of drugs or other chemicals in a patient with hemodynamic and/or neurological impairment.

Instrumental data may reveal serious acute conditions such as cerebral vascular bleeding, contusion or subarachnoid hemorrhage with impaired consciousness or focal neurological signs with at least one vital function deficiency; rupture of bladder, liver, uterus, or esophageal varices with hemodynamic instability after surgical treatment or when there are no indications for treatment [5].

Lastly, pathologies such as myocardial infarction with complex arrhythmias, hemodynamic instability, congestive heart failure with respiratory failure or total heart block with hemodynamic instability must be accompanied by respiratory failure to access in ICU rather than in coronary units.

For selecting patients for intensive care, different scores and models have been proposed.

Physiological severity scoring, in particular the Acute Physiology and Chronic Health Evaluation (APACHE) system, was a transformational concept, introduced as a tool to characterize patient populations and to inform decision-making about individual patients. Physician experience may be a valuable tool for contextualizing population-based prognostic estimates for individual patients [6].

The priority of access to intensive care is managed according to a well-standardized model approved by all scientific companies in the sector (Table 7.1).

Table 7.1 ICU admission prioritization framework [7]

Level of care	Priority	Type of patient
ICU	Priority 1	Critically ill patients who require life support for organ failure, intensive monitoring, and therapies only provided in the ICU environment. Life support includes invasive ventilation, continuous renal replacement therapies, invasive hemodynamic monitoring to direct aggressive hemodynamic interventions, extracorporeal membrane oxygenation, intraaortic balloon pumps, and other situations requiring critical care (e.g., patients with severe hypoxemia or in shock)
	Priority 2	Patients, as described above, with significantly lower probability of recovery and who would like to receive intensive care therapies but not cardiopulmonary resuscitation in case of cardiac arrest (e.g., patients with metastatic cancer and respiratory failure secondary to pneumonia or in septic shock requiring vasopressors)
IMU	Priority 3	Patients with organ dysfunction who require intensive monitoring and/ or therapies (e.g., noninvasive ventilation), or who, m the clinical opinion of the triaging physician, could be managed at a lower level of care than the ICU (e.g., postoperative patients who require close monitoring for risk of deterioration or require intense postoperative care, patients with respiratory insufficiency tolerating intermittent noninvasive ventilation). These patients may need to be admitted to the ICU if early management fails to prevent deterioration or there is no IMU capability in the hospital
	Priority 4	Patients, as described above but with lower probability of recovery/ survival (e.g, patients with underlying metastatic disease) who do not want to be intubated or resuscitated. As above, if the hospital does not have IMU capability, these patients could be considered for ICU in special circumstances
Palliative care	Priority 5	Terminal or moribund patients with no possibility of recovery, such patients are in general not appropriate for ICU admission (unless they are potential organ donors). In cases in which individuals have unequivocally declined intensive care therapies or have irreversible processes such as metastatic cancer with no additional chemotherapy or radiation therapy options, palliative care should be initially offered

IMU Intermediate medical unit

The above considerations, about screening and access to ICU, represent the cornerstone of the management of intensive care in a usual contest of twenty-first century.

Pandemic crisis, like Sars-CoV2, open completely different settings.

7.1.2 The Guidelines During COVID-19 Epidemy

In the previous guidelines three models for guiding admission were discussed: the prioritization model, the diagnosis model, and the objective parameters model. In the prioritization model, patients are categorized by four priority levels based on how likely they are to benefit from admission to the ICU. In the diagnosis model, a list of specific conditions and diseases is offered for deciding which patients should be admitted to the ICU. In the objective parameters model, specific vital signs, laboratory values, imaging or electrocardiogram findings, and physical findings are offered for deciding which patients should be admitted. All these models have limitations, and none have been properly validated [8].

There is high likelihood that the number of critically ill patients will overwhelm hospital systems during the COVID-19 epidemic.

When a regional health system is no longer able to care for an overwhelming number of critically ill patients, a triage plan is necessary to ensure the greatest benefit to the greatest number, and to reduce the number of patients who will be unable to receive critical care resources.

There is a need to ensure that patients who do not initially receive critical care resources are still provided the best supportive care possible and are re-evaluated, at minimum daily, for consideration of resource allocation as supplies become available. This will result in a sliding scale from crisis to contingency and flexibility should be anticipated.

Triage systems should apply to all critically ill patients during pandemics, not solely to those afflicted by COVID-19. Triage decisions should be made by a dedicated triage team, distinct from the primary team providing bedside care.

The American College of Chest Physicians proposed a triage model for the ICU based on three essential steps [9]. In this model the physician must assess whether the patient presents criteria for access to intensive care, whether in agreement (if possible) and whether this option can improve the prognosis of the patient based on individualized clinical and epidemiological criteria (Fig. 7.1).

Without a triage plan, patients will receive critical care resources by random chance or a first-come, first-serve basis, likely leading to overall worse outcomes across a population and more individuals being denied critical care.

Then, the best available epidemiological data, combined with expert input, will be required to create triage protocols that reflect COVID-19-specific mortality and resource utilization predictions.

Although the use of acute illness scores, such as the Sequential Organ Failure Assessment (SOFA) score, was proposed for the previous pandemic triage plans but evidence suggests such scoring systems are unlikely to predict critical care

Triage Decision Algorithm

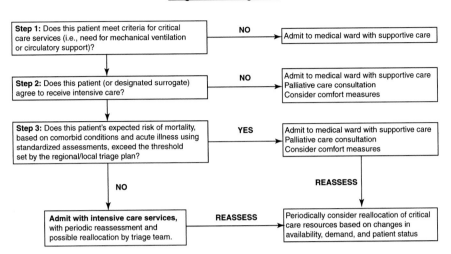

Fig. 7.1 Triage decision process flow proposed by American College of Chest Physicians [9]

outcomes with sufficient accuracy in particular patients suffering from COVID-19 [10].

If the pandemic stretches resources beyond the ability to care for all patients, some states have developed plans to use a SOFA score > 11 as a cutoff to help with decision-making in these dire situations. However, recent studies have shown that SOFA should be used cautiously as part of a decision-making framework and does not meet the ethical cutoffs for prediction across different patient populations [11].

For patients presenting to the emergency department with CAP (Community Acquired Pneumonia), it has been established that delayed admission to the ICU is associated with higher mortality. The **SMART-COP** score was designed to predict which patients with CAP require intensive respiratory or vasopressor support. It uses readily available information, and is 92.3% sensitive in identifying which patients need ICU-level care. In contrast to other scores, SMART-COP does not explicitly consider age as a variable, although it does include age-adjusted cutoffs for respiratory rate and oxygen level [12].

The **SCAP score** uses eight variables that identify patients at risk for "severe CAP," defined by adverse outcomes such as need for ICU admission, development of sepsis, or requirement of mechanical ventilation. SMART-COP and SCAP share several common predictors of adverse patient-oriented outcomes potentially necessitating a higher level of care: age (SMART-COP, aged >50 years; SCAP aged >80 years), multilobar involvement on radiography, respiratory rate >30 breaths/min, confusion (new onset), $PaO_2/FiO_2 < 250$ mmHg, decreased pH (SMART-COP, <7.35; SCAP, <7.30), and systolic blood pressure < 90 mmHg [13].

From the Italian experience during the COVID epidemic there is also a score, **The BCRSS/algorithm**. It uses patient examination features along with the need for escalating levels of respiratory support (noninvasive ventilation, intubation, proning) to suggest treatment recommendations. The scale has not been validated or tested in other populations and was developed as the world continued to learn more about COVID-19 each day [14].

Neither of these elements can be evaluated separately to make decisions regarding the management of the COVID-19 patient but they can be valuable tools in framing patients with borderline ICU access criteria [15].

In support of an adequate organizational level and the epidemiological evaluation of its resources, it has been necessary to divide patients into appropriate categories:

- **Paucisymptomatic COVID patients or level 1**, with flu-like syndrome and without concomitant pathologies such as to require hospitalization; they are kept at home with active health surveillance.
- **COVID patients with moderate respiratory symptoms or level 2**, can be directed to well-equipped hospital wards or SICU, where they can receive NIV and medium-advanced monitoring.

  The criteria for selecting patients to receive NIV include clinical indicators of acute respiratory failure such as dyspnea, tachypnea, the use of accessory respiratory muscles, paradoxical breathing, and disorders in gas exchange.

  This information can be supplemented by imaging, US thorax and EGA.

  Monitoring the patient using the same tools must recognize the failure of NIV as early as possible.

  The severity of respiratory acidosis can be a starting point for identifying patients who may benefit from NIV or require more intensive assistance.

  A pH <7.20, a PaO_2/FiO_2 ratio <100 or <175 after 1 h of NIV, and a SAPS score > 34 are parameters that alone can require the transfer to ICU for ARDS due to COVID-19 [16].

  Unstable hemodynamic conditions, severe bleeding of the upper gastrointestinal tract, incoercible vomiting, undrained PNX, inability to protect the airways, and serious neurologic conditions such as coma or seizures are contraindications to the use of NIV which in case of related COVID IRA require an invasive ventilation.

  Anyway, the hospital management of a COVID patient should be carried out by expert personal in a protected environment where it is possible to quickly shift towards more complex assistance.
- **COVID patients with significant respiratory symptoms, or with significant comorbidities or level 3** (dialyzed, immunocompromised) intended for immediate access to the ICU.

  Patients with pH <7.10 fall into this category; severe hypoxemia $PaO_2/FiO_2 < 100$, strong hemodynamic impairment with the need for vasopressors, severe MOF associated and/or with SAPS score > 34 and all categories of patients with absolute contraindications to NIV.
- **Non-COVID patients with medium-severe respiratory symptoms** who are referred through local services to hospitals no COVID, when possible and compatible with the clinical contest.

Patients with criteria for ICU admission while waiting for the outcome of the swab must temporally stay in appropriate areas, expressly identified, where isolation must be guaranteed [17].

7.2   Conclusion

Triage systems should apply to all critically ill patients during pandemics, not solely to those afflicted by COVID-19. Triage decisions should be made by a dedicated triage team, distinct from the primary team providing bedside care.

References

1. Manca D. Analysis of the number growth of ICU patients with Covid-19 in Italy and Lombardy updated to 17-march, day #25 evening; ESA journal march 18th, 2020.
2. Wunsch H, Linde-Zwirble W, Harrison D, Barnato AE, Rowan KM, Angus DC. Use of intensive care services during terminal hospitalizations in England and the United States. Am J Respir Crit Care Med. 2009;180:875–80.
3. Institute of Medicine. Crossing the quality chasm: a new health system for the 21st century. Washington, DC: The National Academies Press; 2001.
4. Gruppo di Studio Ad Hoc della Commissione di Bioetica della SIAARTI. SIAARTI guidelines for admission to and discharge from Intensive Care Units and for the limitation of treatment in intensive care. Minerva Anestesiol. 2003;69:101.
5. Kim JE, Lee S. Intensive care unit admission protocol controlled by intensivists can reduce transfer delays from the emergency department in critically ill patients. Hong Kong J Emerg Med. 2019;26(2):84–90.
6. Bion J, Dennis A. Oxford text book critical care (ed. 2): ICU admission and discharge criteria. Oxford: Oxford University Press; 2016.
7. Nates JL. ICU admission, discharge, and triage guidelines: a framework to enhance clinical operations, development of institutional policies, and further research. Crit Care Med. 2016;44(8):1553–602.
8. Task Force of the American College of Critical Care Medicine, Society of Critical Care Medcine. Guidelines for intensive care unit admission, discharge, and triage Task Force of the American College of Critical Care Medicine, Society of Critical Care Medicine. Crit Care Med. 1999;27:633–8.
9. Maves RC, et al. Triage of scarce critical care resources in COVID-19: an implementation guide for regional allocation: an expert panel report of the task force for mass critical care and the American College of Chest Physicians. Chest. 2020;158:212–25.
10. Cheung WK, Myburgh J, Seppelt IM, et al. A multicentre evaluation of two intensive care unit triage protocols for use in an influenza pandemic. Med J Aust. 2012;197(3):178–81.
11. United States Department of Health and Human Services. "Topic collection: crisis standards of care." Accessed 17 Mar 2020.
12. Charles PG, Wolfe R, Whitby M, et al. SMART-COP: a tool for predicting the need for intensive respiratory or vasopressor support in community-acquired pneumonia. Clin Infect Dis. 2008;47(3):375–84.
13. España PP, Capelastegui AM, Gorordo I, et al. Development and validation of a clinical prediction rule for severe community-acquired pneumonia. Am J Respir Crit Care Med. 2006;174(11):1249–56.
14. Duca A, et al. Calculated decisions: Brescia-COVID respiratory severity scale (BCRSS)/algorithm. Emerg Med Pract. 2020;22(5 Suppl):CD1–2.

15. Giwa A, Desai A, Duca A. Novel 2019 coronavirus SARS-CoV-2 (COVID-19): an updated overview for emergency clinicians. Emerg Med Pract. 2020;22(5):1–28.
16. Antonelli M, Conti G, Esquinas A, et al. A multiple-center survey on the use in clinical practice of non-invasive ventilation as first-line intervention for acute respiratory distress syndrome. Crit Care Med. 2007;35:18–35.
17. Landini, Belardinelli et al., Linee di indirizzo per la gestione del percorso COVID-19 in ambito ospedaliero e peri-ospedaliero della regione Toscana. April 2020.

The Decision-Making Process of Selection in the Clinical Pathway for COVID-19: The Recommendations for Older Patients

8

Andrea Fabbo, Marilena De Guglielmo, and Andrea Spanò

8.1 Introduction

The COVID-19 pandemic is impacting the global population in dramatic and widespread ways. In all countries, the elderly people are the most exposed to the disease and the most "frail" because of the life challenges imposed by the pandemic status. Although all age groups are at risk of contracting COVID-19, older people are at a higher risk of severe illness and death from the COVID-19 disease due to physiological changes of ageing and potential underlying health conditions [1, 2]. The WHO has reported that over 95% of deaths due to COVID-19 in Europe have been 60 years or older, and more than 50% of all fatalities involved people aged 80 years or older. Reports show that 8 out of 10 deaths are occurring in individuals with at least one comorbidity, in particular those with cardiovascular disease, hypertension and diabetes, but also with a range of other chronic underlying conditions [3, 4]. Public discourses and current opinions about COVID-19 highlight that it is a disease of older people which can lead to social stigma and exacerbate negative stereotypes about ageing. Social stigma in the context of this pandemic crisis and the

A. Fabbo (✉)
Geriatric Service, Cognitive Disorders and Dementia Unit, Health Authority and Services (AUSL) of Modena, Modena, Italy
e-mail: a.fabbo@ausl.mo.it

M. De Guglielmo
Pneumological Service, Primary Care Department, Health Authority and Services (AUSL) of Modena, Modena, Italy
e-mail: m.deguglielmo@ausl.mo.it

A. Spanò
Medical Director of the Modena City District, Health Authority and Services (AUSL) of Modena, Modena, Italy
e-mail: a.spano@ausl.mo.it

© The Editor(s) (if applicable) and The Author(s), under exclusive license to Springer Nature Switzerland AG 2020
N. Vargas, A. M. Esquinas (eds.), *Covid-19 Airway Management and Ventilation Strategy for Critically Ill Older Patients*, https://doi.org/10.1007/978-3-030-55621-1_8

possible limitation of healthcare resources can result in discrimination against older people, a different type of care or exclusion from the most appropriate and specific treatment for that case or situation [5]. The Madrid International Plan of Action on Ageing identifies barriers to healthcare services. It evaluates that older people can experience age-based discrimination in healthcare settings when treatments are considered less important than younger people [6]. So during the pandemic crisis due to COVID-19, international human rights experts warned that clinical decisions regarding the use of intensive care or support such as ventilators could be influenced only by the age criterion and not by other factors related to the overall and functional health status [7]. There is also a strong appeal to governments to develop and follow evidence-based guidelines and recommendations to ensure that medical decisions are based on medical need, ethical criteria and the best available scientific evidence. In the last years, there has been an increase in the elderly population admitted to the intensive care unit (ICU) and the proportion of the very old (85 years or over) critically ill patients is very high especially during the COVID-19 crisis [8]. It cannot be denied that the care of older patients often determines ethical and practical challenges both before and during admission to intensive care [9]. This decision-making process requires some skills like remarkable knowledge of ageing and its consequences on the normal function of organs, competence in comprehensive geriatric assessment and good communication ability with the family and other caregivers [10]. In this chapter, we will discuss the decision-making process of selection in the clinical pathway for COVID-19 dedicated to elderly patients from the triage to admission in intensive care to discharge, an acute or long-term care (in hospital or Long Term Care Facility) or palliative care.

8.2 The Geriatric Assessment

A general assessment of functional status is essential for older patients. The level of physical dependence is measured through validated rating scales such as ADL (Activities of Daily Living) and IADL (Instrumental Activities of Daily Living) [11, 12]. Still, also it represents a milestone in the definition of "frailty". The "frailty model" includes some areas such as biological and physiological function, comorbidity, functional impairment and social vulnerability. Furthermore, all these elements are present in the CGA. An example of a GCA tool is Multidimensional Prognostic Index (MPI) that could be used to evaluate high-risk older patient predicting the risk level (low, moderate or severe) of all-cause mortality, especially in hospital settings. This tool (based on some crucial indicators of CGA such as nutritional status, physical activity, mobility, strength, cognition and mood and social support) would seem to be an accurate predictor of short- and long-term all-cause mortality, length of stay and clinical evolution of older patient admitted in hospital [13]. A recent study compared the accuracy of some geriatric health indicators in predicting different outcomes such as mortality and hospitalisation: one of these, in addition to CFS (or frailty index), frailty phenotype (FP), walking speed and multimorbidity, is HAT (Health Assessment Tool), a summary score including clinical diagnoses, functioning and disability [14]. HAT evaluates five characteristics: walking speed, Mini-Mental State Examination (MMSE) score, difficulties in instrumental activities of daily living (IADL), limitations in basic activities of daily living (ADL) and list of chronic diseases obtaining a score ranging from 0 (poor health) to 10 (good health) [15]. Therefore, the clinical approach to the older patient, from the admission to the hospital, should consider these variables and have the possibility to use a validated approach that assesses the frailty and all the typical aspects of the "geriatric" patient. This occurs using when it is possible, the framework of comprehensive geriatric assessment (CGA) which has been shown (compared with usual care) to improve the chances of persons being alive 1 year later hospitalisation [16]. As there is often a mismatch between the clinicians' assessment and the patient's wishes, multidisciplinary collaboration in the decision-making process is strongly recommended especially for the very old because all healthcare providers who can help to improve the decision-making process for the benefit of the patient should be involved [17].

8.3 The Decision-Making Process for an Older Patient

The COVID-19 pandemic poses urgent questions: older age and the presence of comorbidities are associated with increased risk of mortality, and the high prevalence of functional and cognitive impairment with behavioural symptoms adds to the risk complexity factors that affect the outcomes and quality of treatments. Elderly people who have comorbidities and need admission to hospital with COVID-19 (because of their difficulty in breathing and the appearance of low oxygen levels) are least likely to benefit from going into the hospital since their admission [18]. Because older patients have multiple comorbidities and high level of frailty, the mortality rate from COVID-19 infection will be high. Early reports suggest the case fatality rate for those over 80, is over 15% [19]. A Chinese study that compared the COVID-19 symptoms in young and older people showed that "fever" was less frequent in older people. There was no difference for cough, asthenia, or digestive signs [20]. At the same time, a French study observed more atypical symptoms and signs such as falls, diarrhoea, renal or liver impairment and delirium probably indicative of greater severity of the disease in this population. Comorbidities or pre-existing frailty could influence the frequency of these signs in older people with COVID-19 infection [21]. A recent narrative review published by an Italian geriatric research group that described the clinical evolution and management approach of COVID-19 disease in the older patient hypothesised the presence of four different phases with peculiar characteristics of symptoms and signs, therapeutic strategies and care settings: a phase one dominated by the "viral response" with respiratory and gastrointestinal symptoms that can be treated at home with hydroxychloroquine and antiviral therapy; a phase two or "pulmonary phase" in which fever and dyspnoea worsen and a rapid diagnosis by a CT scan and hospitalisation is required; a phase three or "pulmonary and hyperinflammatory phase", clinically represented by acute respiratory distress syndrome (ARDS) managed in sub-intensive wards and treated with corticosteroids and IL-6 receptor antagonists; a phase four or "vasculitic-thrombotic phase" characterised by pulmonary thrombosis and abnormal D-dimer increase in which anticoagulant therapy should be introduced in addition to admission in ICU indicated in this very critical phase [22]. All previous phases of the COVID-infection can be complicated by the presence of bacterial over-infection: therefore, supportive and specific antibiotic therapy should always be prescribed [23]. Another study noted that dyspnoea, lymphocytopenia, comorbidities (including cardiovascular disease and chronic obstructive pulmonary disease) and acute respiratory distress syndrome were predictive of poor outcome with rapid disease progress observed in mortality reports with a median survival time of 5 days after admission in hospital [24]. Therefore in an older patient with multimorbidity, the COVID-19 illness could have a more serious course; despite hospitalisation and intensive care, mortality in this group is very high: in the experience of intensive-care specialists working in a critical area, very few mechanically ventilated elderly patients with acute respiratory distress syndrome (ARDS) survive [25]. For this reason, the question of whether hospitalisation is indicated for older patients with COVID-19 with multimorbidity should be carefully evaluated; it may be appropriate only in case of concomitant complications of the disease. Moreover, most people would prefer to die not in an intensive care unit, but in a family and "friendly" environment. Consequently, planning of care should be crucial before or at the latest when the infection is diagnosed. An emerging issue is the management of elderly patients with cognitive impairment and respiratory failure due to COVID-19, which requires hospitalisation. Although some studies showed a better management of symptoms in very elderly hospitalised patients in a geriatric ward with the involvement of family caregiver and the attention to the quality of life [26], this condition is very difficult to implement during an extraordinary situation such as the Coronavirus outbreak. Public health emergencies require clinicians to change their practice to respond to the care needs of populations. The shift from "patient-centred practice" to patient care guided by public health duties creates great tension for clinicians because of contrast between the "duty of care " (focus on the individual patient) whose goal is to maintain fidelity to the patient, relieve suffering, respect the rights and preferences of patients and "duties of public health" that recognise moral equality of persons, promote equity in the distribution of risks and benefits, promote public safety, protect community health and fairly allocate limited resources. During pandemics, the ethical imperatives shift: we must consider the safety of not only the individual patient but also the protection of clinicians, the real clinical needs of the population and the effective availability of intensive resources. For example, guidelines on attempting cardiopulmonary resuscitation (CPR) [27] or Clinical Ethics Recommendations for the Allocation of Intensive Care Treatments in exceptional, resource-limited circumstances published by SIAARTI (Italian Society of Anesthesia, Analgesia, Resuscitation and Intensive Care) in the acute hospital setting for patients with COVID-19 have produced conflict and moral discomfort because of differences of opinion about the balance of benefits, the need of treatments and care for everyone and risks to both patients and staff [28]. Special attention should be paid to some vulnerable populations because of particular risks/

burdens that these groups may incur during a pandemic event; this is not necessarily it means they deserve special or different treatment, but we should think about how these groups can be managed according to appropriateness and quality of care. The elderly are often at higher risk of severe disease in times of PLEID (Potentially Lethal Emerging Infectious Diseases); therefore advance directives should be explored in this group to guarantee older patients are participating in decision-making with respect of wishes and respect to outcomes of treatments within the limits of this dramatic event [29, 30]. Multidisciplinary collaboration in the decision-making process is strongly recommended [17], and it provides several important aspects like interdisciplinary reflection, mutual respect in the team, the culture of not avoiding of end-life decisions, active involves of nurses in decision-making and good communication skills. In our clinical practice of geriatricians working in various settings during the COVID-19 emergency in Italy (Hospital or Long Term Care Facility), we performed an evaluation procedure (based on literature recommendations and clinical guidelines) which can be used both at hospital admission and in the long-term care facility to identify the best pathway in hospital settings or avoid unnecessary hospitalisation. The decision-making on whether to send an elderly with certain or suspected COVID-19 disease to hospital requires an assessment based on the principles of proportionality and appropriateness of the treatment, which is based on the knowledge of the following factors:

1. Health indicators (clinical, functional and cognitive status)
2. Prognosis
3. Practical expected benefits of intensive intervention

This evaluation, which falls within the concept of "advance care planning ", must also include a possible knowledge of patient's wishes and a comparison with the family members since, if the evaluation, sharing and communication process are hesitant in the condition of not hospitalising, palliative interventions will be implemented necessary to ensure the best possible care (in terms of dignity and quality of life) for the older patient in this emergency phase. The National Institute for Health and Care Excellence (NICE) guidelines (COVID-19 rapid guideline: critical care in adults published for the management of the pandemic by COVID-19 on 20.03.2020) allow identifying the levels of frailty using the CFS (Clinical Frailty Scale) tool, as part of a global and comprehensive assessment available on the NHS Specialized Clinical Frailty Network website [31, 32]. The use of the CFS is based on a clinical evaluation conducted by an expert geriatrician together with the healthcare providers team (general practitioners, nurse, specialist) based on medical history, drugs, social history, physical disabilities or functional limitations, mobility and use of aids, cognitive status, comorbidity which are collected in a checklist (see Table 8.1) that includes four variables:

1. Global health status: ongoing problems, fitness level, drugs
2. Presence and absence of any active disease (comorbidity assessment performed by Cumulative Illness Rating Scale-CIRS) [33]

Table 8.1 Checklist for assessment of frailty and decision-making in the clinical pathway of the older patient

Name		
Age (score)		
Gender	M	F
Ongoing problems (to describe)		
Drugs (number and list)		
Comorbidity CIRS (score)		
Autonomy ADL (score)		
Cognitive status MMSE (score)		
CFS (score)		
Informed consent	Yes	No
Advanced directives	Yes	No
Surrogate (or administrator)	Yes	No
Share with family	Yes	No
Critical care	Yes	No
Hospital care	Yes	No
Palliative care	Yes	No

3. Level of dependence in the activities of daily living (Katz index) [11]
4. Cognitive state (Mini-Mental State Examination- MMSE) [34]

The goal of the CFS is to identify patients who are at high risk of "intervention failure" and inappropriate treatment in an intensive hospital-type environment (critical, semi-intensive, intensive area). Evaluation with the CFS requires that:

1. If the person has a score lower than or equal to 5, he is likely to receive a benefit from intensive treatment in a hospital or a critical area.
2. If the person has a score higher than 5, it is expected that he will not receive benefit from intensive care treatment but from treatments aimed at improving the clinical condition or controlling symptoms or limiting the discomfort (palliative care).

The use of the tool allows assessing frailty both when the older patient is admitted to the hospital (during the triage phase) and when he is in a nursing home or in another setting to decide if he must be hospitalised before triage admission. So it is possible to organise the most appropriate care interventions by limiting the inconvenience of elderly, family members and care team.

It is important to plan in advance in case an older patient develops symptoms of COVID-19 that get worse. Thus to support decision-making for patients, families and public, it is essential to reflect on issues such as: How will intensive care treatments help the person in the short and long term? Intensive care treatments may offer an acceptable quality of life for the person? Could ICU treatments help to achieve the patient's goals for a good life? Are there non-critical treatments that can help the person and be more comfortable for them? What are the wishes of the individual towards the end-of-life care? The position paper of Alzheimer's Disease International "COVID-19 and dementia: difficult decisions about hospital admission and triage" invites families of elderly people living with dementia to consider developing advance care plan or directives to ensure that patient's wishes are considered when they develop the disease or when they are admitted in the hospital. Moreover, the paper remembers that the health system should provide access to palliative care services in a very care setting (hospitals, nursing home, home care) for persons critically ill with COVID-19 who can choose (or help to choose) not to be hospitalised or to be admitted in critical care by their wishes to avoid suffering, or who have a poor prognosis even if they were admitted to intensive care [35]. Although advanced directives should be available for older patients, very often in "real world" healthcare directives have not been discussed before admission in clinical pathways such as critical care, acute care, long-term care or palliative care. In general, any access to a clinical pathway or treatment requires informed consent from the concerned person. "Informed consent" in medicine is the process by which a patient agrees to a procedure or a treatment. Informed consent is strongly related to the assessment of the patient's decision-making capacity (DMC) for treatment, and there is a strong relationship between the ability to make decisions and cognitive status. There are many causes frequently associated with cognitive impairment in older patients, including the presence of delirium, acute illnesses or dementia that can influence decision-making [36]. Among the few instruments existing in the literature to evaluate the capacity to provide informant consent, the most used is the MacArthur Competence Assessment Tool-Treatment (MacCAT-T) used in subjects with cognitive deficits or impaired mental state [37]; this tool is influenced by the MMSE and it assesses the four dimensions related to competence to consent to treatment: understanding relevant information, appreciation (patient ability to acknowledge the disease or a specific problem), rationalisation (assesses patient ability to reason about treatment options, risks and benefits of treatment/research and consequences of treatment) and communication (capacity to express a treatment choice). Recently the possibility of routine use of MacCAT-T in older people was discussed before beginning a programme of end-of-life care and showed that this tool for clinical research and treatment has the most empirical support [38]. We consider some possibilities: (a) the older patient has a normal cognitive status and can consent to care; usually such conversation should be conducted in the presence of the family or caregivers; (b) when the older patient is unable to consent to care, physicians should discuss the intensity and level of care with the surrogate decision-maker (family member or caregivers); the question is not what the surrogate think about care (for example intensive care or palliative care), but what they know about patient's wishes and how the patient would have responded; (c) in emergencies such as COVID-19 crisis, there is no time for information retrieval from family or caregivers and treatments are usually started without informed consent. In many countries, life-prolonging therapies can be suspended when information is available. Many studies have shown better management in an older patient hospitalised in a non-intensive care unit setting followed by a multidisciplinary team conforming to principles of CGA (comprehensive geriatric assessment), the involvement of surrogate (family caregiver) and the attention to the quality of life. On the other hand, the family members of older patients (with or without dementia) in critical illness play an essential role in the decision-making process relating to treatment and for the physicians may be difficult to know the patient's wishes and preferences despite that Italian Law on informed consent provided by a supporting administrator and advance directives (DAT) has been approved [39, 40]. Family members of older incompetent patients are increasingly playing an essential role in the decision-making process relating to medical treatment or clinical pathway; a recent European review regarding surrogacy laws for an older patient with limited decision-making capacity have identified two main essential issues in the absence of the advance directives: the role of family members automatically accepted as surrogates by law and a legal representative appointed by a court. The necessity of a legal representative (as it happens in Italian legal system) is a common position in many European member states. The possibility that the physicians could decide without informed consent is possible only in a few countries (such as the UK) if it is in the best interest of the patient and corresponds to his wishes [41]. Like any critical illness, the COVID-19 disease causes significant psychosocial stress to the patient, family members and surrogates due to fear and anxiety about the infection, high-level isolation precautions including visitation limitation or the inability to assist loved ones at the end of life. The importance to discuss end-of-life wishes with older patients and their family should occur early (perhaps even before a potential diagnosis), especially if conditions of "high frailty" and comorbidity are already known and that have a poor prognosis in case they develop acute respiratory distress syndrome (ARDS) or other complications. If so, a consultation with the palliative care team should be done to assist the elderly and families in decision-making and assist clinicians on issues that may arise about appropriate treatments and procedures. Patients who are currently followed by palliative care teams will, in general, not be eligible for intensive care treatment in the case of a COVID-19 infection. This is also true for most older patients in nursing homes, according to our protocol (see checklist described above) or international guidelines. It is important to document the patients' wishes and the presence of advance directives already established and make the documents available for an acute situation [42–44]. Particularly in the cases of absence of anticipating directives already formulated, an "individual care plan" (PAI) is configured as the only adequate instrument to prepare an accompanying shared path. The PAI identifies the acts of care and assistance that the multidisciplinary team considers ethical and appropriate to pursue and must be understood as a flexible instrument whose objectives are subject to periodic verification and adjustment. This approach to the end-of-life phase is particularly important. The European Association of Palliative Care (EAPC) has drafted a consensus statement trying to define some practical principles to use along the path of caring for people at the end of life. Great emphasis is given to anticipate directives as a dynamic process of reflection and dialogue between the person, his/her family members and health professionals regarding preferences for care and assistance [45].

8.4   Conclusive Remarks

The pandemic of coronavirus disease of 2019 (COVID-19) has a global impact not only on the health system but also on the economic and social aspects of daily life that are changing rapidly. The groups most susceptible to COVID-19 are older adults and those with chronic underlying medical problems or very vulnerable conditions such as loneliness or cognitive and psychiatric disorders. The Geriatric scientific societies have emphasised that despite the presence of a good health system in some national contexts, despite timely warnings and even documented indications to pay attention to the older adults and vulnerable population, the COVID-19 pandemic found us largely unprepared [46, 47]. And once again, the emergency showed us that the elderly paid the highest costs in terms of higher attack rates, suffering and mortality. The population residing in long-term care facilities are generally more exposed both because they are older and with greater comorbidities and because the organisation often is not adequate to respond to such serious health emergencies. The clinical evolution and the pathophysiology of the COVID-19 disease especially in an older patient require skills and adaptability in a clinical context that can change rapidly, and that raises endless questions in terms of achievable objectives and appropriateness of care. This has important clinical and ethical implications in the hospital and community care. It is, therefore, necessary to consider older patients' likelihood of surviving to hospital discharge, assessed with an evaluation of acute illness severity, and older patient's likelihood of longer-term survival based on an assessment of comorbid conditions that can influence survival [48].

8.5   Recommendations

1. An approach based on comprehensive geriatric assessment (CGA) and the identification of levels of "frailty" becomes essential in the decision-making process to guarantee the most appropriate levels of care both in a critical area and in the long-term or palliative care in accordance, when it is possible, with the wishes and individual needs of the older patient.
2. In the hospital or long-term facility the physicians cannot avoid providing an organisation based on person-centred care that collects, respect wishes and individual needs. Hence they should promote advanced directives also a thorough evaluation of decision-making capacity (involving the patient or the surrogate) which can be influenced by pathological changes of mental status or cognitive impairment often present in this vulnerable population.
3. The mission of Geriatrics is to identify and to treat older patients maximally benefiting of goal-oriented, tailored, multidisciplinary interventions and to identify patients at risk of poor outcomes such as the "very frail" elderly to guarantee the best possible quality of life and avoid unnecessary treatment. Older people have the same rights to be cared for as younger people.
4. Triage must be done on clinical appropriateness and not on personal age or other characteristics such as disability.

5. A position paper by the European Geriatric Medicine Society (EUGMS) suggests that advanced age should not itself be a criterion for excluding patients from hospital care settings (intensive and otherwise) than outside the hospital [49].

6. Innovative and simplified models of comprehensive geriatric assessment (CGA) and tailored and validated interventions of geriatric medicine (including evaluation of frailty, cognitive status, hydration and nutritional, prevention of adverse events related to drugs and psychosocial support) are the guidelines needed to ensure appropriate interventions in older patients. These models should be applied in every care setting from primary care to hospital and Long Term Care facility.

7. When no benefit of treatments can be obtained, palliative care should be considered. The decision to hospitalise requires an evaluation inspired by the principles of proportionality and appropriateness of the treatment, which includes the assessment of the overall conditions (clinical, functional, cognitive) including prognosis and realistic expected benefits of intensive intervention.

8. The intensive care is therapy not suitable for people who start from a situation of high fragility due to pre-existing severe pathologies and in any case to a poor functional reserve with a risk of damage (due to the pathology and the necessary intensive manoeuvres) more remarkable than the expected benefits. A reflection as early as possible that avoids a treatment path determined by hasty decisions based only on the management of the symptom (however serious), and aimed at defining/sharing the level of adequacy of the treatments available, accompanied when possible by advanced directives, could allow older people to be treated and die in a context of care consistent with their real chances of therapeutic success.

9. If the evaluation and comparison with a family member or surrogate hesitate in the decision not to hospitalise, the palliative interventions necessary to control the disturbing symptoms and suffering and to guarantee comfort will be implemented.

10. "Older persons have faced higher infection and mortality rates, while at the same time being subjected to ageism in public discourse, age discrimination in health care and triage decisions, neglect and domestic abuse at home, isolation without access to essential services, and greater exposure and poor treatment in care institutions" according to United Nations Policy on Human Rights [50].

"Older persons have faced higher infection and mortality rates, while at the same time being subjected to ageism in public discourse, age discrimination in health care and triage decisions, neglect and domestic abuse at home, isolation without access to essential services, and greater exposure and poor treatment in care institutions" according to United Nations Policy on Human Rights [79].

"My inspiration and my passion will always come from my older patients. One day I hope to be like them; when that day comes, I hope that my doctor will be a geriatrician."
William R, Hazzard WR, "I am a Geriatrician"; 2004
Hazzard WR. I am a Geriatrician. J Am Geriatr Soc 2004;52:161.

References

1. Onder G, Rezza G, Brusaferro S. Case-fatality rate and characteristics of patients dying in relation to COVID-19 in Italy. JAMA. 2020;323:1775–6. https://doi.org/10.1001/jama.2020.4683.
2. WHO "Coronavirus disease 2019-Situation Report 51". 2020.
3. Grasselli G, Zangrillo A, Zanella A, et al. Baseline characteristics and outcomes of 1591 patients infected with SARS-CoV-2 admitted to ICUs of the Lombardy region, Italy. JAMA. 2020;323:1574–81. https://doi.org/10.1001/jama.2020.5394.
4. Zhou F, Yu T, Du R, Fan G, Liu Y, Liu Z, Xiang J, Wang Y, Song B, Gu X, Guan L, Wei Y, Li H, Wu X, Xu J, Tu S, Zhang Y, Chen H, Cao B. Clinical course and risk factors for mortality of adult inpatients with COVID-19 in Wuhan, China: a retrospective cohort study. Lancet. 2020;395(10229):1054–62. https://doi.org/10.1016/S0140-6736(20)30566-3.
5. IFRC, UNICEF. WHO "Social Stigma associated with COVID-19". 2020.
6. Political Declaration and Madrid International Plan of Action on Ageing, Second World Assembly on Ageing, Madrid, Spain, 8–12 April, 2002 https://www.un.org/en/events/pastevents/pdfs/Madrid_plan.pdf.
7. "Unacceptable"—UN expert urges better protection of older persons facing the highest risk of the COVID-19 pandemic, United Nations Human Rights, Geneva, March 27, 2020. https://www.ohchr.org/EN/NewsEvents/Pages/DisplayNews.
8. Flaatten H, de Lange DW, Artigas A, Bin D, Moreno R, Christensen S, et al. The status of intensive care medicine research and a future agenda for very old patients in the ICU. Intensive Care Med. 2017;43(9):1319–28.
9. Leblanc G, Boumendil A, Guidet B. Ten things to know about critically ill elderly patients. Intensive Care Med. 2017;43(2):217–9.
10. Guidet B, Vallet H, Boddaert J, et al. Caring for the critically ill patients over 80: a narrative review. Ann Intensive Care. 2018;8:114. https://doi.org/10.1186/s13613-018-0458-7.
11. Katz S, Akpom CA. 12. Index of ADL. Med Care. 1976;14(5 Suppl):116–8.
12. Lawton MP, Brody EM. Assessment of older people: self-maintaining and instrumental activities of daily living. The Gerontologist. 1969;9(3):179–86.
13. Pilotto A, Cella A, Pilotto A, et al. Three decades of comprehensive geriatric assessment evidence coming from different healthcare settings and specific clinical conditions. J Am Med Dir Assoc. 2017;18(2):192.e1–e11.
14. Zucchelli A, Vetrano DL, Grande G, et al. Comparing the prognostic value of geriatric health indicators: a population-based study. BMC Med. 2019;17:185. https://doi.org/10.1186/s12916-019-1418-2.
15. Santoni G, Marengoni A, Calderón-Larrañaga A, Angleman S, Rizzuto D, Welmer AK, Mangialasche F, Orsini N, Fratiglioni L. Defining health trajectories in older adults with five clinical indicators. J Gerontol A Biol Sci Med Sci. 2017;72(8):1123–9.
16. Ellis G, Gardner M, Tsiachristas A, et al. Comprehensive geriatric assessment for older adults admitted to hospital. Cochrane Data base Syst Rev. 2017;9:CD006211. https://doi.org/10.1002/14651858.CD006211.pub3.
17. Van den Bulcke B, Piers R, Jensen HI, Malmgren J, Metaxa V, Reyners AK, et al. Ethical decision-making climate in the ICU: theoretical framework and validation of a self-assessment tool. BMJ Qual Saf. 2018;27(10):781–9.
18. Wu Z, McGoogan JM. Characteristics of and important lessons from the coronavirus disease 2019 (COVID-19) outbreak in China: summary of a report of 72 314 cases from the Chinese Center for Disease Control and Prevention. JAMA. 2020;323(13):1239–42. https://doi.org/10.1001/jama.2020.2648.
19. D'Adamo H, Yoshikawa T, Ouslander JG. Coronavirus disease 2019 in geriatrics and long-term care: the ABCDs of COVID-19. J Am Geriatr Soc. 2020;68:912–7. https://doi.org/10.1111/jgs.16445.
20. Liu K, Chen Y, Lin R, Han K. Clinical features of COVID-19 in elderly patients: a comparison with young and middle-aged patients. J Inf Secur. 2020;80(6):e14–8. https://doi.org/10.1016/j.jinf.2020.03.005.

21. Godaert L, Proye E, Demoustier-Tampere D, Coulibaly PS, Hequet F, Dramé M. Clinical characteristics of older patients: the experience of a geriatric short-stay unit dedicated to patients with COVID-19 in France. J Inf Secur. 2020;81:e93–4. https://doi.org/10.1016/j.jinf.2020.04.009.

22. Lauretani F, Ravazzoni G, Roberti MF, Longobucco Y, Adorni E, Grossi M, De Iorio A, La Porta U, Fazio C, Gallini E, Federici R, Salvi M, Ciarrocchi E, Rossi F, Bergamin M, Bussolati G, Grieco I, Broccoli F, Zucchini I, Ielo G, Morganti S, Artoni A, Arisi A, Tagliaferri S, Maggio M. Assessment and treatment of older individuals with COVID 19 multi-system disease: clinical and ethical implications. Acta Bio Med. 2020;91(2):1. https://www.mattioli1885journals.com/index.php/actabiomedica/article/view/9629

23. Jin YH, Cai L, Cheng ZS, et al. A rapid advice guideline for the diagnosis and treatment of 2019 novel coronavirus (2019-nCoV) infected pneumonia (standard version). Mil Med Res. 2020;7(1):4.

24. Wang L, He W, Yu X, Hu D, Bao M, Liu H, Zhou J, Jiang H. Coronavirus disease 2019 in elderly patients: characteristics and prognostic factors based on 4-week follow-up. J Inf Secur. 2020;80:639–45. https://doi.org/10.1016/j.jinf.2020.03.019.

25. Bouadma L, Lescure F, Lucet J, et al. Severe SARS-CoV-2 infections: practical considerations and management strategy for intensivists. Intensive Care Med. 2020;46:579. https://doi.org/10.1007/s00134-020-05967-x.

26. Ahmed NN, Pearce SE. Acute care for the elderly: a literature review. Populat Health Manag. 2010;13(4):219–25. https://doi.org/10.1089/pop.2009.0058.

27. Fritz Z, Gavin D. Perkins cardiopulmonary resuscitation after hospital admission with Covid-19 the balance of benefits and risks has changed, and practice must change with it. BMJ. 2020;369:m1387. https://doi.org/10.1136/bmj.m1387.

28. Vergano M, Bertolini G, Giannini A, et al. Clinical ethics recommendations for the allocation of intensive care treatments in exceptional, resource-limited circumstances: the Italian perspective during the COVID-19 epidemic. Crit Care. 2020;24:165. https://doi.org/10.1186/s13054-020-02891-w.

29. Berlinger N. Ethical framework for health care institutions responding to novel coronavirus SARS-CoV-2 (COVID-19). Guidelines for Institutional Ethics Services Responding to COVID-19. The Hastings Center–March 16, 2020. https://snlg.iss.it/wp-content/uploads/2020/03/AA-Hastings-Center-Covid-Framework-2020.pdf.

30. Hick JL, Hanfling D, Wynia MK, Pavia AT. Duty to plan: health care, crisis standards of care, and novel coronavirus SARS-CoV-S. In: NAM Perspectives. Discussion paper. Washington, DC: National Academy of Medicine; 2020.

31. COVID-19 rapid guideline: critical care in adults NICE guideline Published: 20 March 2020. www.nice.org.uk/guidance/ng159.

32. NHS Specialised Clinical Frailty Network (https://www.scfn.org.uk/clinical-frailty-scale).

33. Miller MD, Paradis CF, Houck PR, Mazumdar S, Stack JA, Rifai AH, Mulsant B, Reynolds CF. Rating chronic medical illness burden in geropsychiatric practice and research: application of the cumulative illness rating scale. Psychiatry Res. 1992;41(3):237–48.

34. Folstein MF, Folstein SE, McHugh PR. 'Mini-Mental State'. A practical method for grading the cognitive state of patients for the clinician. J Psychiatr Res. 1975;12:189–98.

35. Alzheimer's Disease International (ADI) position paper: COVID-19 and dementia: Difficult decisions about hospital admission and triage, 9 April 2020. https://www.alz.co.uk/news/adi-releases-position-paper-on-covid-19-and-dementia.

36. Fabbo A. Legal issues (surrogacy laws, informed consent). In: Esquinas AM, Vargas N, editors. Ventilatory support and oxygen therapy in elder, palliative and end-of-life care patients. Berlin: Springer; 2019. p. 325–38. https://doi.org/10.1007/978-3-030-26664-6_37.

37. Santos RL, Sousa MF, Neto SJP, Bertrand E, Mograbi DC, Landeira-Fernandez J, Laks J, Dourado MC. MacArthur competence assessment tool for treatment in Alzheimer disease: cross-cultural adaptation. Arq Neuropsiquiatr. 2017;75:36–43.

38. Kiriaev O, Chacko E, Jurgens JD, Ramages M, Malpas P, Cheung G. Should capacity assessments be performed routinely prior to discussing advance care planning with older people? Int

Psychogeriatr. 2018; 16:1–8. Tate JA, Sereika S, Divirgilio D. et al Symptom communication during critical illness: the impact of age, delirium and delirium presentation. J Gerontol Nurs. 2013;39:28–38.

39. Legge 22 dicembre 2017 n.219 Norme in materia di consenso informato e di disposizioni anticipate di trattamento (GU Repubblica Italiana Serie Generale n.12 del 16.01.2018).

40. Di Luca A, et al. Law on advance health care directives: a medical perspective. La Clinica Terapeutica. 2018;169(2):e77–81. https://www.clinicaterapeutica.it/ojs/index.php/ClinicaTerapeutica/article/view/150.

41. Tibullo L, Esquinas AM, Vargas M, Fabbo A, Micillo F, Parisi A, Vargas N. Who gets to decide for the older patient with a limited decision-making capacity: a review of surrogacy laws in the European Union. Eur Geriatr Med. 2018;9:759–69. https://doi.org/10.1007/s41999-018-0121-8.

42. Roland K. Minder Markus COVID-19 pandemic: palliative care for elderly and frail patients at home and in residential and nursing homes. Zurich/Berlin/Vienna, approved by the Board of the Association for Geriatric Palliative Medicine (FGPG) (www.fgpg.eu) on 22 March 2020. Swiss Med Wkly. 2020;150:w20235. https://doi.org/10.4414/smw.2020.20235.

43. Lovell N, Maddock M, Etkind SN, Taylor K, Carey I, Vora V, Marsh L, Higginson IJ, Prentice W, Edmonds P, Sleeman KE. Characteristics, symptom management and outcomes of 101 patients with COVID-19 referred for hospital palliative care. J Pain Symptom Manag. 2020;60:E77–81. https://doi.org/10.1016/j.jpainsymman.2020.04.015.

44. Fusi-Schmidhauser T, Treston N, Keller N, Gamondi C. Conservative management of Covid-19 patients–emergency palliative care in action. J Pain Symptom Manag. 2020;60:e27. https://doi.org/10.1016/j.jpainsymman.2020.03.030.

45. van der Steen JT, et al. on behalf of the European Association for Palliative Care (EAPC). White paper defining optimal palliative care in older people with dementia: A Delphi study and recommendations from the European Association for Palliative Care. Palliat Med. 2014;28(3):197–209.

46. Polidori MC, Maggi S, Mattace-Raso F, Pilotto A. The unavoidable costs of frailty: a geriatric perspective in the time of COVID-19. Geriatric Care. 2020;6(1):1. https://doi.org/10.4081/gc.2020.8989.

47. Kimball, A, Harfield, KM, Arons, M, James, A, Taylor, J, Spicer, K, et al. Asymptomatic and presymptomatic SARS-CoV-2 infections in residents of a long-term care skilled nursing facility—King County, Washington, March 2020. Centers for Disease Control MMWR Early Release. Vol. 69, March 27, 2020. https://www.cdc.gov/mmwr/volumes/69/wr/mm6913e1.htm?s_cid=mm6913e1.

48. White DB, Lo B. A framework for rationing ventilators and critical care beds during the COVID-19 pandemic. JAMA. 2020;323:1773–4. https://doi.org/10.1001/jama.2020.5046.

49. EuGMS, European Geriatric Medicine Society. STATEMENT of the EuGMS Executive Board on the COVID-19 epidemic. https://www.eugms.org/fileadmin/user_uploadNews_Documents/News_2020/EuGMS_Statement_on_COVID-19.pdf.

50. United Nations. Policy Brief: The impact of COVID-19 on older persons (May 2020) https://reliefweb.int/report/world/policy-brief-impact-covid-19-older-persons-may-2020.

COVID-19: End-of-Life Care Decision-Making and Preferences in Older People

9

Nicola Vargas, Adriano Palmieri, and Antonio M. Esquinas

9.1 Introduction

Elderly patients, frail, and with underlying many chronic comorbidities or severe illness are most at risk from COVID-19 pandemic. Recent data from the Italian Istituto Superiore di Sanità (ISS) showed that COVID-19 is more lethal in older subjects. In Italy, on the date of March 17, 2020, the overall case-fatality rate was 7.2%, and 96.4% of died patients had more than 60 years. When age groups stratified data, individuals aged 70 years or older represent 35.5% of cases, while subjects aged ≥80 years were 52.3% [1]. With respect to the severe context of widespread world mortality, the main aims of the palliative care (quality of life, discernment of patient goals, advance care planning, pain and symptom management, and support for caregivers over protracted trajectories) may appear not essential [2]. The COVID-19 pandemic showed, conversely, the limits of the healthcare system on managing elderly patient's wishes even and expectations during the dreadful COVID-19 disease. During epidemic such as that of SARS CoV 2, the necessity of intensive care unit (ICU) beds could be not sufficient for the patients with severe respiratory distress (ARDS). Many recommendations suggest, in these contests, that the physicians should guarantee the healthcare resources to the patients with a higher life expectancy. The evaluation for the need for intensive care should include the severity of the disease, the comorbidity and the presence of multi-organ failure. Have besides, in this period, the patient's

N. Vargas (✉) · A. Palmieri
Department of Medicine, Geriatric and Intensive Geriatric Ward, San Giuseppe Moscati Hospital, Avellino, Italy

A. M. Esquinas
Intensive Care Unit, Hospital Morales Meseguer, Murcia, Spain

N. Vargas, A. M. Esquinas (eds.), *Covid-19 Airway Management and Ventilation Strategy for Critically Ill Older Patients*, https://doi.org/10.1007/978-3-030-55621-1_9

wishes, advance care planning and even end of life preference a central value? This chapter would analyse this prerogative in light of the severity of COVID pandemic.

9.2   The Unexpected Scenario of COVID-19 Disease and Older Patients

During COVID-19 pandemic, many older patients, with a chronic life-limiting illness, may have a rapid change of own health status. They switched from the condition of chronic patients to an unexpected end-of-life scenario. A new fast assessment of older patient's goals and wishes is necessary. Many factors play a role in changing the caring plans with new health events (Table 9.1). Hospital management for COVID disease prohibited family and authorised representatives to visit acutely and chronically ill older patients [2]. Family members no longer play the role of direct participation in the decision-making process for their loved ones. Sometimes they have no notice about the health state of their parents. Family members often only apprehended of their death. Abruptly they lose the central role of caregiver and experience emotional distance. Elderly competent patients may live in a deep state of isolation. Furthermore, some external (not dependent on patients or their family background) factors influence the decision-making process in critically ill older patients. The acute respiratory failure, for example, necessitates, during the pandemic, to have ventilators and ICU beds sufficient. If they are in a low number, hospitals will propose alternative care not included in advance directives. But, if the patients have an advance directive or advance care planning the triage and physicians' choice will be more comfortable. In the case of the absence of these directives, the physicians may select the patients according to age and life expectancy as suggested by scientific society [3]. Besides, even in the COVID period, the wishes of patients can be challenging to determine because of their uncertainty about what they want, cognitive impairment, personal and cultural barriers to the articulation of their preferences, and competing preferences of patients and relatives [4]. During severe acute illness, the oldest old patients, even when they are competent, are often unable to express their wishes. They may have a passive role in the doctor–patient relationship. Furthermore, older patients usually prefer to defer the decision about intensive cares to others. They frequently prefer that physicians have more significant input in the decision-making process [5]. This rule is still more true for competent older patients who live a sense of social separation, such as during COVID pandemic. During an epidemic,

Table 9.1 Factors that limit the expression of preferences in older patients during COVID-19 pandemic

1. Isolation. Prohibition family and representatives to visit to acutely and chronically ill older patients. Family are advised not to touch or even be in the same room as loved ones
2. Quickly deterioration with no sufficient time to discuss an advance care planning
3. Physicians' overworking and burnout
4. Scientific society recommendations with exclusion of older patients from intensive care

the time may be short when patients deteriorate quickly, separation is mandated, and families are advised not to touch or even be in the same room as loved ones [6]. The person-centred care may become very difficult and changing their own planned advance directives too in the light of the new scenario. In this complicated context, physicians have a central role. They represent the closest decision-making level for the family and patients. But, during a pandemic, they are even at the risk of burnout. In general, burnout is a psychological syndrome that involves a prolonged response to chronic interpersonal stressors on the job [7]. In the pandemic period, it is due to the emotional stress, overworking, frustration and impotence towards a severe illness. Physicians often see their colleagues fall ill.

9.3 End-of-Life Preferences of Older Patients: Recommendations During the COVID Pandemic

In the scenario of rationing the resources for some patients, end-of-life care will be viewed as preferable for others because little chance of survival with a meaningful quality of life exists. Advance directives and known individual preferences influence in some patients, this decision [8]. Furthermore, even in the COVID, person-centred care has never been more necessary, including sensitive advance care planning conversations and best interest decisions—communicated clearly with compassion. The physicians should guarantee the symptom control, the support of family and friends from a distance [9]. End-of-life decisions include withholding or withdrawing life-sustaining treatments which deemed non-beneficial for the patients. The patients, even in a condition of precipitating scenario, should continue to take an active role at the end of life. Proper communication with patient and family about the use of NIV, for example, instead of invasive mechanical ventilation, is essential. NIV may be a powerful tool for the relief of breathlessness symptom management [10]. Many elders in their 70s, 80s, 90s and 100s would not want to be put on a respirator if they become critically ill from COVID-19. Patients and our health system would be better served if all adults and elders use some of the spare time created by our new, home-confined lives to discuss and document their care preferences. The absence of such planning increases suffering at the end of life, and its presence helps people with severe or life-limiting illness to live and die according to their priorities [11].

9.4 Conclusion

During a pandemic, the "unexpected" meaning may be a factor that eliminates the active role of older patients at the end of the life decision-making process. Some crucial factors, such as the short availability of ventilators or intensive care beds, may first exclude the possibility that the older patient may make a choice or express his/her preferences. However, during a pandemic, caring based on patients' centred and on care planning, even with family distant is needed.

References

1. Onder G, Rezza G, Brusaferro S. Case fatality rate and characteristics of patients dying in rela-tion to COVID-19 in Italy. JAMA. 2020; https://doi.org/10.1001/jama.2020.4683.
2. Available at https://www.chcf.org/blog/the-role-of-palliative-care-in-a-covid-19-pandemic/.
3. http://www.siaarti.it/SiteAssets/News/COVID19%20%20documenti%20SIAARTI/SIAARTI%20-%20Covid19%20-%20Raccomandazioni%20di%20etica%20clinica.pdf.
4. Rockwood K, Powell C. End-of-life decision-making in community-acquired pneumonia. In: Marrie TJ, editor. Community-acquired pneumonia. Boston, MA: Springer; 2002.
5. Vargas N, Tibullo L, Landi E, et al. Caring for critically ill oldest old patients: a clinical review. Aging Clin Exp Res. 2017;29:833–45. https://doi.org/10.1007/s40520-016-0638-y.
6. For the *Lancet* Commission on Palliative Care and Pain Relief see https://www.thelancet.com/commissions/palliative-care Palliative care and the COVID-19 pandemic www.thelancet.com Vol 395 April 11, 2020 doi:https://doi.org/10.1016/S0140-6736(20)30822-9
7. Maslach C, Leiter MP. New insights into burnout and health care: strategies for improving civility and alleviating burnout. Med Teach. 2017;39(2):160–3.
8. Vincent J-L, Taccone FS. Understanding pathways to death in patients with COVID-19. Lancet Respir Med. 8(5):430–2. https://doi.org/10.1016/S2213-2600(20)30165-X.
9. British Geriatrics Society. COVID-19: End of life care in older people. Available at https://www.bgs.org.uk/resources/covid-19-end-of-life-care-in-older-people.
10. Erdogan E, Dikmen Y. Chapter 36: NIV in palliative mediicne and end-of-life care: the per-spectives of patients, families and cliniccians. In: Esquinas AM, Vargas N, editors. Ventialtory support and oxygen therapy in elder, palliative and end-of-life care patients. New York: Springer Nature; 2020.
11. Aronson L. Age, complexity, and crisis—a prescription for Progress in pandemic. N Engl J Med. 383:4. https://doi.org/10.1056/NEJMp2006115.

Part IV

Management of ARF

The Impact Frailty, Co-morbidity and Ageing of the Respiratory System on the Unfavourable Prognosis of COVID-19

10

Marilena De Guglielmo and Andrea Fabbo

10.1 Introduction

Some of the reasons COVID-19 greatly impacts older people include the physiological changes associated with ageing, decreased immune function, frailty and multimorbidity (Fig. 10.1) which expose older adults to be more susceptible to the infection itself and make them more likely to suffer severely from COVID-19 disease and more severe complications. Older adults are at a significantly increased risk of severe illness following infection from COVID-19. This observation is very significant for the European Region: of the top 30 countries with the largest percentage of older people, all but one (Japan) are our Member States in Europe [1]. A different approach based on comprehensive geriatric assessment (CGA) could help to better identify older patients more at risk of dismal outcomes and who, at some point of their clinical course, will need the ICU admission [2]. The factors to consider in this approach are ageing, co-morbidities, use of drugs, malnutrition, cognitive impairment and functional decline, better known as a condition of "frailty". All of these elements are part of the CGA defined as a process used by healthcare practitioners to assess the status of older people to optimise health management and care [3, 4]. The multidimensional approach is mainly due to the clinical complexity of older patients. They have multiple and interdependent problems which make their care more challenging than in younger people, or those with just one medical

M. De Guglielmo (✉)
Pneumological Service, Primary Care Department, Health Authority and Services (AUSL) of Modena, Modena, Italy
e-mail: m.deguglielmo@ausl.mo.it

A. Fabbo
Geriatric Service, Cognitive Disorders and Dementia Unit, Health Authority and Services (AUSL) of Modena, Modena, Italy

© The Editor(s) (if applicable) and The Author(s), under exclusive license to
Springer Nature Switzerland AG 2020
N. Vargas, A. M. Esquinas (eds.), *Covid-19 Airway Management and Ventilation Strategy for Critically Ill Older Patients*, https://doi.org/10.1007/978-3-030-55621-1_10

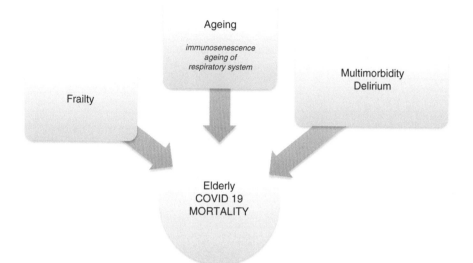

Fig. 10.1 Interdipendent Factors that influence the COVID-19 pneumonia in elderly

problem. In this chapter, the authors analysed all the factors of multidimensional evaluation to assess their impact on the poor prognosis of the elderly viral pneumonia (Fig. 10.1).

10.2 Frailty

Frailty involves a complex interaction of biological, social and cognitive factors that negatively impact an individual's ability to complete their activities of daily living (ADLs) independently. Moreover, "Frailty" represents a greater vulnerability to an acute stressor with consequent difficulty in adapting to them. One of the most used and validated tools to evaluate fragility is the Clinical Frailty Scale [5], which stratifies older patient in nine groups from "very fit" to "terminally ill". An increased CFS is associated with a higher risk of mortality and complications such as falls, reduced mobility and adverse events. A recent meta-analysis shows that an elderly with high CSF values have higher hospitalisation risks and higher mortality in intensive care (ICU) [6] and another European study showed that in critical patients over 80 years with high frailty (CSF > 5) the 30-day mortality in ICU exceeded 30% of cases. Consecutive classes in Clinical Frailty Scale were inversely associated with short-term survival [7]. It is suggested that you can also use faster tools like FRAIL screen (a five-item scale that evaluates fatigue, resistance, ambulation, illnesses and loss of weight) used to detect older persons at increased risk [8]. The use of the clinical phenotypes for identifying the frailty syndrome in the ageing population has gained substantial and significant clinical guidance over the past years. However, geriatric medicine is now being faced with a new worldwide enemy, COVID-19, that together with older age, hypertension and type 2 diabetes may clinically define the "COVID Spiraling Frailty Syndrome" [9]. Frailty has a significant effect on the reduction of functional reserve and on elderly ability to answer appropriately to an acute stressor such as COVID-19 viral pneumonia infection.

10.3 Multimorbidity

Multimorbidity increases in the elderly [10] the proportion of patients with co-morbidities and the number of co-morbidities per patients increase with age. The most common co-morbidities in older people are hypertension, diabetes, chronic obstructive pulmonary disease, cardiac failure, cancer and dementia [11]. Multimorbidity is associated with increased mortality, loss in physical autonomy and an increase in hospitalisation rates and long-term mortality rates, especially in critical care [12]. Ageing and multimorbidity contribute to frailty, which, in turn, confers a higher risk of several complications and poor outcomes such as falls, disability, hospitalisation and mortality [13]. The Charlson co-morbidity index has been validated in critically ill patients and is predictive of mortality [14]. Because of multiple chronic conditions, the elderly patient often uses various medications (polypharmacy) that expose him to a series of adverse events (indicators of frailty) such as falling, hospital admissions and ultimately death [15]. Polypharmacy and inappropriate medications prescription among older patients frequently lead to adverse outcomes; often acute hospitalisations determine an increased risk of the incorrect prescription, the presence of polypharmacy, inadequate medication reconciliation and a lack of care coordination [16]. However, initially, current models of the population mortality impact of COVID-19 are based on age-stratified death rates over days in patients infected with COVID-19. They have not incorporated clinical information from NHS health records regarding the prevalence of underlying conditions. Epidemiological data suggest that multimorbid older patients have the poorest prognosis. However, it is conceivable that age and number of co-morbidities alone do not reflect the real condition and the expected prognosis of the patients affected by COVID-19 [17]. We know that over 95% of these deaths occurred in those older than 60 years. More than 50% of all deaths were people aged 80 years or older. We also know from reports that 8 out of 10 deaths are occurring in individuals with at least one underlying co-morbidity, in particular those with cardiovascular diseases/hypertension and diabetes, but also with a range of other chronic underlying conditions [1]. In Italy, the data about the pre-existing conditions based on 481/3200 patients dying in-hospital (15.0% of the sample) showed that the mean number of diseases was 2.7. Overall, 1.2% of the sample presented with a no co-morbidities, 23.5% with single co-morbidity, 26.6% with 2, and 48.6% with three or more [18]. The COVID infection evidenced in older patients a linear correlation between the number of diseases and mortality rate.

10.4 The Ageing Process

Ageing is a heterogeneous process, with individuals ageing depending on their genetic background, environmental exposures and other factors. Ageing is a complex condition represented by a physiological and cognitive vulnerability, making the person more susceptible to stressor agents (biological, psychological and environmental factors), diseases and acute medical events and causing further reduction in a reserve capacity, loss of functional independence and increased risk of mortality [19]. A component of ageing is the imbalance between inflammatory and anti-inflammatory networks in individuals resulting in a low-grade chronic inflammatory state referred to as "inflammaging", which is a condition characterised by elevated levels of blood inflammatory markers that carry high susceptibility to chronic morbidity, disability, frailty and premature death [20]. The combination of immunosuppression and "inflame-ageing", called "immunosenescence", results in higher rates of viral reactivation and infection susceptibility and severity [21]. The effect of ageing on the entire respiratory system has many structural and functional changes on thoracic cage, lungs and respiratory muscles. Chest wall compliance is reduced by osteoporosis changes with shortening of the thoracic vertebrae. The elastic recoil is decreased significantly, contributing to air trapping. The causes of gas exchange are because of decrease of the total alveolar area, the capillary volume, and the density of pulmonary capillary and the progressive increase of the closing volume (CV) during expiration, which determine the heterogeneity of the ventilation/perfusion ratio within the lungs and reduction of diffusion capacity of the lung for carbon monoxide (DLCO), with the subsequent decline in the $PaCO_2$ and increase of the arteriolar–alveolar gradient (A-a-DO2) [22].

10.5 Cognitive Disorders and Delirium

In critical care, the presence of cognitive impairment is associated with a high risk of delirium that is the most common complication afflicting hospitalised patients age 65 older, even if it often remains unrecognised [23]. Delirium is associated with increased mortality, high length of stay, risk of premature institutionalisation and subsequent further cognitive decline [24]. The American Psychiatric Association's fifth edition of the Diagnostic and Statistical Manual of Mental Disorders (DSM-5) defines delirium as a syndrome characterised by an acute onset and fluctuating course of symptoms such as inattention, impaired level of consciousness and disturbance of cognition (e.g. disorientation, memory impairment, or alteration in language) [25]. The "gold standard" and the most widely used tool for assessing delirium remains the Confusion Assessment Method (CAM) which provides an algorithm based on the four core features of delirium: acute onset, fluctuating course of symptoms, inattention, and either disorganised thinking or altered level of consciousness [26]. Other characteristics that support the diagnosis of delirium are alterations in the sleep-wake rhythm, alterations in perception (e.g. hallucinations), emotional lability, delusions and inappropriate or unsafe behaviours. The CAM algorithm has been validated in research and has high sensitivity (94–100%) and specificity (90–95%) with good interrater reliability. The CAM has also been adapted for use in the ICU, emergency departments, nursing homes, and palliative care. Another exciting and quick tool is the 4AT Test which has been validated in clinical settings involving dementia patients and is easy to administer with good sensitivity (about 90%) [27]. Delirium can be classified into three clinical subtypes: hyperactive (characterised by psychomotor agitation, restlessness, delusions and heightened arousal), hypoactive (characterised by sleepiness, lack of interest in daily activities, and being quiet and withdrawn) or mixed type delirium (represented by the alternation of hyperkinetic and hypokinetic phases). Delirium without agitation occurs in >50% of patients. In the type hypoactive and mixed, it can be more challenging to recognise. Its assessment is essential to consider detectable and treatable risk factors early. Despite the high incidence and prevalence in ICU, delirium is often underdiagnosed, especially hypokinetic delirium. In critical care assessment, it is necessarily carried out in two phases: a first phase that assesses the level of consciousness through a validated scale as The Richmond Agitation Sedation Scale (RASS) [28] and a second phase that evaluates cognitive functioning through CAM-ICU. With deep sedation levels (RASS = −4 or −5) the CAM-ICU scale is not administered, and the patient is described as "not evaluable"; when we have more superficial sedation levels (RASS ≥ −3), you can move on to the second phase. CAM-ICU it is a validated standard scale that can be used daily for the evaluation of the delirium in intensive care [29].

10.6   Conclusion

The negative outcome and increased mortality characterise the COVID-19 pneumonia in the elderly. The reason behind this worst outcome is some prominent factors that are interdependent such as the frailty state, the ageing of the respiratory system, multimorbidity and delirium and cognitive impairment. All these factors influence the outcome and the organisations of ICU management of critical elderly patients. A correct multidimensional approach may include and capture all these aspects.

References

1. Statement–Older people are at highest risk from COVID-19, but all must act to prevent community spread. Dr Hans Henri P. Kluge, WHO Regional Director for Europe. http://www.euro.who.int/en/health-topics/health-emergencies/coronavirus-covid19/statements/statement-older - people – are – at – highest – risk – from – covid – 19,- but-all – must – act – to – prevent – community – spread.
2. Welsh TJ, Gordon AL, Gladman JR. Comprehensive geriatric assessment—a guide for the non-specialist. Int J Clin Pract. 2014;68(3):290–3. https://doi.org/10.1111/ijcp.12313.
3. Rubenstein LZ, Stuck AE. Multidimensional geriatric assessment. In: Pathy's principles and practice of geriatric medicine. New York: Wiley; 2012. p. 1375–86. https://doi.org/10.1002/9781119952930.ch112.

4. National Institutes of Health Consensus Development Conference. Statement: geriatric assessment methods for clinical decision-making. J Am Geriatr Soc. 1988;36:342–7.
5. Rockwood K, Song X, Macknight C, Berman H, Hogan DB, Mcdowell I, Mitnitski A. A global clinical measure of fitness and frailty in elderly people. CMAJ. 2005;173(5):489–95.
6. Muscedere J, Waters B, Varambally A, Bagshaw SM, Boyd JG, Maslove D, et al. The impact of frailty on intensive care unit outcomes: a systematic review and meta-analysis. Intensive Care Med. 2017;43(8):1105–22.
7. Flaatten H, De Lange DW, Morandi A, Andersen FH, Artigas A, Bertolini G, et al. The impact of frailty on ICU and 30-day mortality and the level of care in very elderly patients (≥80 years). Intensive Care Med. 2017;43(12):1820–8.
8. Dent E, Morley JE, Cruz-Jentoft AJ, et al. Physical frailty: ICFSR international clinical practice guidelines for identification and management. J Nutr Health Aging. 2019;23(9):771–87.
9. Abbatecola AM, Antonelli-Incalzi R. COVID-19 spiraling of frailty in older Italian patients. J Nutr Health Aging. 2020;2020:1–3. https://doi.org/10.1007/s12603-020-1357-9.
10. Barnett K, Mercer SW, Norbury M, et al. Epidemiology of multimorbidity and implications for health care, research, and medical education: a cross-sectional study. Lancet. 2012;380:37–43.
11. Salive ME. Multimorbidity in older adults. Epidemiol Rev. 2013;35:75–83.
12. Zampieri FG, Colombari F. The impact of performance status and comorbidities on the short-term prognosis of very elderly patients admitted to the ICU. BMC Anesthesiol. 2014;14:59.
13. Fried LP, Ferrucci L, Darer J, et al. Untangling the concepts of disability, frailty, and comorbidity: implications for improved targeting and care. J Gerontol A Biol Sci Med Sci. 2004;59:255–63.
14. Stavem K, Hoel H, Skjaker SA, Haagensen R. Charlson comorbidity index derived from chart review or administrative data: agreement and prediction of mortality in intensive care patients. Clin Epidemiol. 2017;9:311–20.
15. de Groot MH, van Campen JP, Kosse NM, de Vries OJ, Beijnen JH, Lamoth CJ. The Association of Medication-use and Frailty-Related Factors with gait performance in older patients. PLoS One. 2016;11(2):e0149888. https://doi.org/10.1371/journal.pone.0149888.
16. Page RL, Linnebur SA, Bryant LL, Ruscin JM. Inappropriate prescribing in the hospitalized elderly patient: defining the problem, evaluation tools, and possible solutions. Clin Interv Aging. 2010;5:75–87.
17. Blanco-Reina E, Ariza-Zafra G, Ocaña-Riola R, León-Ortiz M. 2012 American Geriatrics Society beers criteria: enhanced applicability for detecting potentially inappropriate medications in European older adults? A comparison with the screening tool of older Person's potentially inappropriate prescriptions. J Am Geriatr Soc. 2014;62(7):1217–23.
18. Available https://www.epicentro.iss.it/coronavirus/bollettino/Report-COVI2019_20_marzo_eng.pdf.
19. Guidet B, Vallet H, Boddaert J, et al. Caring for the critically ill patients over 80: a narrative review. Ann Intensive Care. 2018;8:114. https://doi.org/10.1186/s13613-018-0458-7.
20. Franceschi C, Capri M, Monti D, et al. Inflammaging and anti-inflammaging: a systemic perspective on aging and longevity emerged from studies in humans. Mech Ageing Dev. 2007;128:92–105.
21. Fulop T, Larbi A, Dupuis G, Le Page A, Frost EH, Cohen AA, Witkowski JM, Franceschi C. Immunosenescence and Inflamm-aging as two sides of the same coin: friends or foes? Front Immunol. 2018;8:1960. https://doi.org/10.3389/fimmu.2017.01960.
22. Romano A, Romano R. Gase xchange and control of breathing in elderly and end-of-life diseases. In: Esquinas AM, Vargas N, editors. Ventilatory support and oxygen therapy in elder, palliative and end-of life care patients. New York: Springer; 2020.
23. Fabbo A, Manni B. Management of elderly patients with delirium syndrome. In: Esquinas AM, Vargas N, editors. Ventilatory support and oxygen therapy in elder, palliative and end-of-life care patients. New York: Springer; 2019. p. 227–39. https://doi.org/10.1007/978-3-030-26664-6_26.
24. Pandharipande PP, Girard TD, Jackson JC, Morandi A, Thompson JL, Pun BT, et al. Long-term cognitive impairment after critical illness. N Engl J Med. 2013;369(14):1306–16.

25. European Delirium Association* and American Delirium Society. The DSM-5 criteria, level of arousal and delirium diagnosis: inclusiveness is safer European Delirium Association. BMC Med. 2014;12:141.
26. Inouye SK, van Dyck CH, Alessi CA, et al. Clarifying confusion: the confusion assessment method: a new method for detection of delirium. Ann Intern Med. 1990;113(12):941–8.
27. Hshieh TT, Inouye SK, Oh ES. Delirium in the elderly. Psychiatr Clin N Am. 2018;41:1–17.
28. Sessler CN, Gosnell MS, Grap MJ, Brophy GM, O'Neal PV, Keane KA, Tesoro EP, Elswick RK. The Richmond agitation-sedation scale: validity and reliability in adult intensive care unit patients. Am J Respir Crit Care Med. 2002 Nov 15;166(10):1338–44.
29. Ely EW, Margolin R, Francis J, May L, Truman B, Dittus B, Speroff T, Gautam S, Bernard G, Inouye S. Evaluation of delirium in critically ill patients: validation of the confusion assessment method for the intensive care unit (CAM-ICU). Crit Care Med. 2001;29:1370–9.

The Physiopathology of COVID Acute Respiratory Failure

Rafael Soler

The current pandemic for the new coronavirus has posed a massive challenge to the scientific community. This new coronavirus (SARS-CoV-2) has surprised professionals so much with its contagiousness and mortality that it has been unexpected.

Most countries have been affected, although unevenly. Millions of people affected worldwide and hundreds of thousands of deaths on the planet are shocking figures for an unknown virus until the end of 2019.

Although the virus affects the entire body, the particular predilection for the respiratory system defines the main complication of this viral affectation, respiratory failure, which, when it appears, does so quickly, between 7 and 10 days after infection.

We know that mortality is practically negligible in children and increases with age, being especially relevant in people over 65 and the elderly. This mortality differs between countries, sometimes very significantly. The different detection strategies of the various countries may probably influence these disparate mortality figures, since the number of tests performed among asymptomatic or oligosymptomatic patients varies widely among countries, since there are countries that have performed tests, (either fast tests or reaction polymerase chain (RPC)), on a massive scale. In contrast, other countries have performed them very selectively, for symptomatic patients. With all these difficulties, we could estimate the actual mortality at around 2–2.50%.

What is clear is that mortality, as we have previously mentioned, increases nonlinearly with age, although this is not the only factor, since the presence of certain comorbidities produces negative synergies with age, in terms of final mortality.

Coronaviruses are enveloped viruses, RNA, with an average size of 30 kb, with a wide variety of host species. There are four main structural proteins: spikes (with

R. Soler (✉)
Department of Neurology, University Hospital, Melilla, Spain

N. Vargas, A. M. Esquinas (eds.), *Covid-19 Airway Management and Ventilation Strategy for Critically Ill Older Patients*, https://doi.org/10.1007/978-3-030-55621-1_11

two essential subunits: S1, responsible for adhesion to the host cell, and S2, whose function is fusion), membrane, envelope and nucleocapsid [1].

There are four main types of coronavirus: alpha, beta, gamma and delta. The alpha types are usually responsible for catarrhal episodes in humans, although SARS-Cov, MERS-CoV (the Middle East Respiratory Syndrome virus) and SARS-CoV-2 are beta coronaviruses [1].

In November 2002, because there was an epidemic of severe pneumonia in Guangdong, China, interest in knowledge about coronaviruses in general significantly increased. SARS is a zoonotic disease. Probably bats are the reservoir host of this virus. Chinese wet-markets sell exotic animals for human consumption and have provided transmission of the virus to man. SARS is spread by close person-to-person contact through droplet transmission or excretions [2].

The Pathology of Severe Acute Respiratory Syndrome in Man demonstrates a variable degree of consolidation, oedema, haemorrhage and congestion of the lungs, and pleural effusion in the thoracic cavity. Diffuse alveolar damage (DAD) is the central fact we can observe in histopathology of SARS.

This stage is related to the duration of the illness, and we observe three stages: an exudative, a proliferative phase and a fibrotic phase.

The exudative phase, the initial 7–10 days, shows necrosis of alveolar epithelial cells, intraluminal oedema, fibrin exudation, hyaline membrane formation, haemorrhage and infiltrates with inflammatory cells into the alveolar wall and lumina, necrosis of the bronchiolar and bronchial epithelium with infiltration of monocytes, lymphocytes and neutrophils into the bronchial wall [2].

In the proliferative phase, after 10–14 days, there is less epithelial damage with interstitial and alveolar fibrosis, bronchiolitis obliterans organizing pneumonia (BOOP), and regeneration that is characterized by pneumocyte hyperplasia. Large multinucleated cells composed of macrophages or pneumocytes are frequent and atypical enlarged pneumocytes with large nuclei, amphophilic granular cytoplasm and prominent nucleoli too.

In the fibrotic phase, after 14 days, interstitial thickening is described with mild to moderate fibrosis and BOOP-like pattern and only a few inflammatory cells (mainly histiocytes and lymphocytes). Other figures are haemophagocytosis, squamous metaplasia and fibrin thrombi in vessels [2].

Although different animal species are susceptible to SARS-CoV infection, we do not have a global animal model to explain the changes.

When we compare the pathological features of SARS in man to the laboratory animal species, there are both similarities and differences.

Firstly, the localization of the lesions is similar among all species: lesions centred on alveoli and bronchioles. Secondly, the character of the lesions is similar among all species; thirdly, the severity of the lesions among species can be divided into two groups, depending on the age. Elderly: severe DAD, characterized by oedema, fibrin and hyaline membranes. Young have milder DAD demonstrating a more multifocal distribution and lacking the above-named features [2].

The development of fibrosis in the late stages of human cases of SARS may be related to several factors: irreversible damage to the pneumocytes, specific epithelial sensitivity to interferon (IFN)-g, and T-helper (Th) 1-dominant immune-mediated cell death. These facts favour the damage to infected alveolar epithelial cells over damage to non-infected fibroblasts, leaving the latter relatively intact. This process leads to the destruction of the epithelial layer, a basis for the stimulation of fibroblasts for repair; there may be Fas-mediated apoptosis of human epithelial cells, while lung fibroblasts are protected and are also not infected by SARS-CoV.

The pathological changes induced by SARS-CoV (in general) infection in man can be related to virus-specific factors and host-specific factors. The virus-specific factors are: receptor specificity, SARS-CoV via the surface spike protein (S-protein) to infect target cells. Several host cell receptors bind to the S-protein: metallopeptidase angiotensin-converting enzyme 2 (ACE2), lectins (C-type lectin DC-SIGN), human CD209L and LSECtin. Binding of the S-protein to the main functional receptor ACE2 on the target cell leads to the fusion between the virus envelope and the host cell membrane.

The central target cells for the virus to infect are epithelial cells of the respiratory tract. The sites of viral replication correspond with the presence of ACE2. Immunohistochemistry studies demonstrate virus antigen or viral nucleic acid in alveolar, bronchiolar, bronchial and tracheal epithelial cells.

Virus-specific factors depend on cytopathic effect, by attachment and infection of the host cells, and attraction of inflammatory cells.

Host-specific factors: immune and inflammatory cells, and induction of cytokines.

The virus and host specific factors can explain the pathogenesis of severe acute respiratory syndrome coronavirus infection in animal models and variation in disease severity in animal models.

Genetic analyses of the host demonstrate that species-to-species variation in the sequence of the ACE2 gene affects the efficiency by which the virus can enter the cells.

Age is another host-specific factor that is related to more severe disease in man. Aged cynomolgus macaque infected with SARS-CoV had more severe lesions than young-adult animals, even though viral replication levels were similar. We have observed similar results in mice: aged mice showed more severe lesions than young-adults, generally indicating a more robust proinflammatory response than in young mice. Age-related accumulated oxidative damage and a weakened anti-oxidative defence system cause a disturbance in the redox balance, resulting in increased reacting oxygen species [2].

The viral life cycle can be summarized in five necessary steps: adherence, penetration, biosynthesis, maturation and release.

Adhesion involves subsequent endocytosis and penetration through the membranes; the final step is the release of the viral RNA into the nucleus of the attacked cell, where the viral RNA replicates, producing new viral proteins, in the process of biosynthesis. When the new particles are mature, they are finally released [1].

Angiotensin-converting enzyme 2 (ACE2) has been identified as a functional receptor for SARS-CoV, and also for SARS-CoV-2 (this is a crucial fact). This receptor is expressed primarily in the lung, heart, intestine, kidney and urinary bladder.

SARS-CoV-2 has unique features, such as the existence of furin cleavage site ("RPPA" sequence) at the S1/S2 site, in a total contrast to SARS-CoV spike (without cleavage). The ubiquitous expression of furin makes this virus very pathogenic.

The symptomatology of SARS-CoV-2 infected patients is highly variable, ranging from asymptomatic or minimally symptomatic patients to severe respiratory failure with multi-organ failure. On the computerized tomography (CT) scan, the characteristic pulmonary ground-glass opacification can be seen even in asymptomatic patients.

We have observed significant ACE2 receptor expression in the apical region of lung epithelial cells in the alveolar space. This item can explain the invasion of the virus and the eventual massive cell destruction. It would also justify early pulmonary involvement of the distal airway.

The inherent immunity of the airway has three main components: epithelial cells, alveolar macrophages and dendritic cells. T cell mediated responses against coronaviruses are of particular relevance. The primary mechanism is usually phagocytosis of the virus-infected epithelial cells. This phagocytosis is carried out by dendritic cells and macrophages, which mediate antigen presentation to T cells [1].

Other mechanisms are the specific adhesion of SARS-CoV to molecule-3-grabbing nonintegrin (DC-SIGN) and DC-SIGN-related protein (DC-SIGNR, L-SIGN). Alveolar macrophages are also directly affected. T cells play a significant role, both CD4+ and CD8+. CD4+ cells produce the activation of virus-specific antibodies; CD8+ T cells can directly attack virus-infected cells, producing cell destruction [1].

When we have carried out immunological studies, mainly in patients with severe affectation, we have observed significant lymphopenia, mainly at the expense of peripheral T cells. Also, we have found high plasma concentrations of proinflammatory cytokines, mainly interleukins (IL), type IL-6 and IL-10; also granulocyte colony-stimulating factors (G-CSF), monocyte chemoattractant protein 1 (MCP1), macrophage inflammatory protein (MIP) 1α, and tumour necrosis factor (TNF)-α.

There is a proportional linear relationship between the disease severity and circulating levels of IL-6. Activation of CD4+ and CD8+ results in higher expression of CD69, CD38 and CD44. T cells are exhausted, reflecting in the levels of Tm3+ PD-1+ receptor subsets in CD4+ and CD8+ T or NK group 2 member A (NKG2A) [1].

This physiopathological T cell debacle may be related to the progression of the disease as well as the appearance of aberrant pathogenic CD4+ T cells.

Another contrasting phenomenon is the production of IL-8, in addition to IL-6, as a result of viral infection of lung epithelial cells. Interleukin-8 is a chemoattractant for neutrophils and T cells, which contributes to lung damage.

Neutrophils play a critical role in this immune storm, directly damaging the lung.

Inflammatory CD14+ and CD16+ monocytes hardly appear in healthy patients but are significantly increased in COVID-19 patients. This fact leads to a significant expression of IL-6, which accelerates the progression of the systemic inflammatory response [1].

ACE2 is widely represented in innate lymphoid cells (ILC) 2 and ILC3. NK cells are a member of ILC1, highly present in the lung. ILC2 and ILC3 are related to mucous homeostasis. The role they play in the pathophysiology of COVID-19 lung damage is unclear.

Acute respiratory failure is the final expression of a complex process.

After recognition of CoVs nucleic acids or proteins, the activation of these sensors generally leads to the activation of the transcription factors IFN-regulatory factor 3 and NF-κB, which stimulate the expression and secretion of Type-I IFN and pro-inflammatory cytokines [3].

The JAK-STAT (Janus kinase/signal transducers and activators of transcription) signalling cascade is activated, leading to the expression of various antiviral interferon-stimulated genes (ISGs) resulting in an antiviral state of the infected cells.

This aspect is associated with the endoplasmic reticulum (ER) stress. When the ER's capacity for folding and processing proteins exceeds, unfolded or misfolded proteins rapidly accumulate in the lumen. This feature leads to the activation of unfolded protein response (UPR) pathways through the induction of protein kinase RNA-like endoplasmic reticulum kinase (PERK), increasing the level of phosphorylated eukaryotic initiation factor 2 alpha (eIF2α), resulting in the promotion of a pro-adaptive signalling pathway by the inhibition of global protein synthesis and selective translation of activating transcription factor 4 (ATF4), inducing pro-apoptotic genes, and a failure of synthesis of anti-apoptotic Bcl-2 proteins.

The ER stress-mediated leakage of calcium into the cytoplasm also leads to the activation of apoptosis effectors.

The viruses, on the other hand, have evolved strategies to suppress and overcome the immune responses, which influence the pathogenesis, course of the disease and persistence of the virus in the host.

The CoVs strategically counteract PKR-mediated signalling to prevent the translational shut-off due to eIF2α phosphorylation. The S proteins (SARS-CoV and SARS-CoV-2) interact with eIF3F, to modulate host translation, including the expression of the pro-inflammatory cytokines, and IL-6 and 8 at a later stage of infection. These interactions play an essential regulatory role in CoV pathogenesis. The hCoV manipulates the translation machinery through nsps. The nsp1 protein, an inhibitor at multiple steps of translation, inhibits 48S initiation complex formation and its conversion into the 80S initiation complex, apart from directly binding to the 40S ribosomal subunit to stall translation [3].

The nsp1 and 40S complex induce cleavage of cellular mRNAs to suppress the translation. The overexpression of the SARS-CoV 3a protein leads to G1 arrest and inhibition of cell proliferation. SARS-CoV infection decreases p53 expression related to antiviral effect and able to enhance its replication in the cells lacking p53 depleted cells.

On the other hand, the protein-protein interactions (PIP) play an essential role. During the viral invasion and infection, both the agent and cellular proteins are continually competing for binding. These interactions, in virus-host systems, are mediated by domain-domain interactions (DDIs). In the case of viral infection, the virus-host PIPs, the interacting proteins are continually stimulating their binding sites in order to evade or optimize interspecific PPIs. The exogenous interfaces lend competition for such molecular reactions and interfere with host–host protein interactions leading to severe alterations in cellular metabolism [3].

Finally, the immune response/inflammasome activation: The SARS-CoV-infected peripheral blood mononuclear cells lead to the upregulation of expression of various cytokines, including IL-8 and IL-17, and the activation of macrophages and the coagulation pathways.

The protein kinases control a wide variety of cellular processes, linked to cellular immune responses, like interleukin (IL) signalling, IL-6 and -8, occurring downregulation of a large number of mRNAs, including those encoding proteins involved in translation, leading to the host translational shut-off in CoV-infected cells. Besides, the heterogeneous nuclear ribonucleoproteins (hnRNPs) influence the maturation of nascent nuclear RNAs into messenger RNAs (mRNAs) and stabilize their cellular transport and control their translation. The immune and inflammatory response determines the outcome of the infection and is responsible for activation of transcription 3 (STAT3) pathways, involved in lung inflammation and cellular repair.

The CoV nucleocapsid (N) protein plays a multifunctional role in the virus life cycle, from the regulation of replication and transcription to genome packaging and release of VLPs to modulation of host cell defence processes.

The viruses encode proteins to modulate the cellular factors to modify the immune response. The RNA viruses, including CoVs, appear to exploit autophagy for the viral replication and propagation.

In the severely ill SARS-CoV-2 patients, the pulmonary disease may progress rapidly to acute respiratory failure. The neutrophil-to-lymphocyte ratio (NLR) is as an independent risk factor for severe illness in these patients. The patients with age ≥ 50 and NLR ≥ 3.13 denote a severe illness and usually need respiratory support. The pyroptosis, a form of inflammatory form of programmed cell death, appears to be the possible mechanism for the increased virulence of SARS [3].

The SARS-CoV Viroporin 3a triggers the activation of the NLRP3 inflammasome and the secretion of IL-1β by macrophages, suggesting SARS-CoV induced cell pyroptosis. These patients have increased IL-1β in the serum, an indicator of the pyroptosis, especially in lymphocytes.

Not only do we talk about purely respiratory symptoms in COVID-19 pulmonary disease, but the lung damage is due to vascular phenomena, such as thrombosis or pulmonary embolism, which occur in patients suffering the most severe conditions. There is a substrate of hypercoagulability in these cases, as demonstrated by the high levels of D-dimer or fibrinogen in the most severe patients, where endothelial damage is relevant, affecting the vasodilatory, fibrinolytic and antiaggregate function of the latter. The expression of endothelial ACE2 plays an unclear role. Likewise, the exceptionally high proportion of endothelial cells in the lung, which represents more than one-third of the cell mass, probably plays a role in the physiopathology of the disease, especially in the most severe cases. Endothelial damage affects microvascular permeability, contributing to facilitate viral invasion [1].

There are physiopathological differences between pulmonary involvement of children and adults or the elderly. Although they are not known precisely, we are progressively having more information about these differential facts.

We know that children tend to have a lower viral load in cases of COVID-19, concerning adults or the elderly. This fact differs significantly from that found in other respiratory viruses, where the opposite is true (respiratory syncytial virus and influenza virus).

The exact cause of this difference in viral loads is not known, although there are several hypotheses.

Firstly, the expression of ACE2 is much higher in adults and older people than in children, as lung tissue and epithelial cells continue to increase and develop from birth, so expression advances with age. The ACE2 gene, located on the X chromosome, may influence the higher levels of ACE2 found in males. Although not confirmed, it may explain some of the fact that mortality is higher in men than in women.

Functional aspects may be important. In this sense, ageing related to continuous antigenic stimulation and thymic involution; this could justify a functional change in T cells, from naïve T cells to central memory T cells, effector and effector memory T cells, and loss of expression of co-stimulatory molecules (CD27, CD28). These phenomena could explain an increased susceptibility to infection.

Also, in children, there is a certain CD4+ and CD8+ immaturity, so the production of inflammatory and cytotoxic mediators is more reduced, as well as less harmful capacity of T cells. This pathogenetic aspect may explain the immune storm, occurring in the most severe cases, is always much lower in children than in adults, and in the latter than in the elderly. Since this storm is considered key in the respiratory and systemic deterioration of the most severe patients, it could explain, in part, why the affectation depends on age, as this mechanism is immature in children. These phenomena have already been demonstrated in experimental animals, mainly monkeys and mice [1].

As age increases, these hyperinflammatory mechanisms are more accentuated and finally condition deterioration in the patient, due to a multisystemic affectation, being the basis of respiratory failure and acute respiratory failure.

Another hypothesis considers the possibility of biological competition. This item means that other viral agents are frequently present in the pulmonary and respiratory tract mucosa in children. This circumstance, according to some authors, could produce a competition phenomenon, which would translate into a lower viral load of COVID-19 [1].

Older adults not only are more susceptible to COVID-19, but they are at significantly increased risk for morbidity and mortality. Infections in this population often present atypically, making it difficult the correct diagnoses. Contributing prognosis factors are physiologic changes and multiple age-related comorbid conditions such as pulmonary and heart diseases, diabetes, and dementia. Most of these patients have associated polypharmacy [4].

The diagnosis is not easy, usually. Although fever is the most common symptom, sometimes fever response is often blunted in older people. It is persistent to observe impaired mobility, falls, confusion, and exacerbation of heart failure in this population, as initial symptoms of ARF.

Coronaviruses have TLR7, RIG-I/MDA, and cGAS/STING innate immune sensors. These sensors influence in early IFN-I responses. Neutralizing antibodies directed at the spike (S) protein binding site for the ACE2 receptor is key to protection, although the much higher affinity of SARS-2 S protein for ACE2 (relative to SARS-1) may pose a challenge [4].

The immune system of older people undergoes many age-related changes (immune senescence). This involution makes the elderly especially vulnerable to new infectious diseases, such as SARS-CoV-2. The main changes we see in ageing are the drop in the production of new T cells due to thymic atrophy, the dysfunction of the bone marrow (later), causing a fall in production of naïve B cells, the involution of lymph nodes (losing naïve T cells and interacting), and dysregulation in chemokines that guide T cell migration. Besides, immune responses do not effectively switch from innate to adaptive (little to no antibody production) [4].

Ageing implies not only a different physiopathology but also a different response to treatments (less effective and more toxic) and a different response to vaccination (under investigation), as the ageing-related immune defects drastically reduce this responsiveness. Immune responses in older adults are slower, less coordinated, and less efficient, making older adults more susceptible to emerging infections.

Diffuse pulmonary endothelial dysfunction is not the only mechanism by which COVID-19 causes respiratory failure. Vascular mechanism is also fundamental: pulmonary microthrombi and significant pulmonary vascular are frequent is these patients. The coexistence of obliterative lesions and vasodilatory regions could explain, on the one hand, the combined dead-space and shunt physiology, and on the other side, the preserved pulmonary haemodynamics and normal right ventricular function reported previously [5].

The improvement in oxygenation related to increased PEEP in this population is due to decreased cardiac output, and decreased shunt fraction rather than to alveolar recruitment.

Our knowledge from the SARS-CoV-1 outbreak (pulmonary thrombi, pulmonary infarcts, and microthrombi in other organs) is not that different than SARS-CoV-2, because pathophysiological aspects are similar.

Microthrombi are present in sepsis and classic forms of ARDS. However, the fundamental cause of respiratory failure is not vascular. However, in COVID-19 acute respiratory failure (ARF), the vascular component may play a different role in gas exchange abnormalities and multisystem organ dysfunction. The preserved lung compliance noted early in patients with bilateral airspace opacities suggests that the observed pulmonary infiltrates could represent areas of pulmonary infarct and haemorrhage [5].

As we have seen previously, older adults are more affected than children by COVID-19. However, there are several factors that make children more affected by respiratory viruses: less competent immune system, far fewer memory cells in the arsenal of children's immune system, shorter bronchial tree making viruses reach alveoli and preventive measures along with personal hygiene usually lower in children.

So what makes COVID-19 infection different from the usual trend of other respiratory viruses? Maybe the immune response is different, especially in ARF. Most of the damage to lung tissue in severe cases is due to severe inflammation rather than a direct damaging effect of the virus itself. So COVIF-19 acts probably very similarly to SARS-CoV-1. In the 2003 SARS outbreak, no single person under the age of 24 has died. It seems that COVID-19 has the same pathogenic effect as SARS 2003 [6].

In severe cases of SARS, the patients, after an initial respiratory phase (fever and cough), while the virus was rapidly replicating in their lungs, usually improved (initial immune response), but the second phase would be much worse than the first, not because of the virus, but because of patients' runaway immune systems.

We do not know the final reasons, but older adults are not able to turn off their inflammatory response, leading immune cells and inflammation-inducing molecules (not only cytokines) to flood into the lungs (cytokine storm). It means a devastating attack on the virally infected cells, and this is exerted by binding neutralizing antibodies to the crown-like spikes of the virus, killing them.

Although we do not know the exact sequence and mechanism, maybe the explanation would be the following one: first, the healthy adults have intact innate immunity along with competent humoral and cell-mediated immunity, so their immune system can limit the infection from progression, preventing the virus from reaching alveoli, and set out recovery within 2–3 weeks from the beginning of symptoms. Second, elderly patients (or weakened patients: co-morbidities, compromised immunity, etc.) do not have the same fit innate and adaptive humoral immune response as healthy adults; therefore, COVID-19 get lower, in huge numbers, until reaching alveoli. Here immune system becomes more aggressive (the last location before virus invades blood circulation). Alveolar lymphocytes and macrophages abundantly guard alveoli. Also, airway epithelial cells act as immune effector, secrete cytokines, chemokines and other factors. This process leads to severe and devastating alveolar and interstitial inflammation (damage of lung tissue and filling alveoli with inflammatory exudates). This item eventually results in severe hypoxia and respiratory failure and may be collateral damage in downstream organs like liver and kidney. Children are less capable of mounting a devastating and vigorous cell-mediated attack on alveoli and interstitial tissue of the lung, maybe due to immature immune system, perhaps due to the lack of adults-like memory cells specific to other circulating coronaviruses [6].

ARF is a life-threatening lung condition that prevents enough oxygen from getting to the lungs and into the circulation. In fatal cases of human SARS-CoV-2 infections, individuals exhibit severe respiratory distress requiring mechanical ventilation, and the histopathology findings also support ARDS. More than 40 candidate genes, including ACE2, interleukin 10 (IL-10), tumour necrosis factor (TNF), and vascular endothelial growth factor (VEGF) are associated with ARF. Increased levels of plasma IL-6 and IL-8 are related to adverse outcomes of ARDS [7].

Cytokine Storm after rapid viral replication and cellular damage, virus-induced ACE2 downregulation and antibody-dependent enhancement (ADE) are responsible for aggressive inflammation caused by COVID-19.

The initial onset of rapid viral replication causes massive epithelial and endothelial cell death and vascular leakage, triggering the production of pro-inflammatory cytokines and chemokines.

Loss of pulmonary ACE2 function is related to acute lung injury (ACE2 downregulation and shedding can lead to dysfunction of the renin-angiotensin system), and further enhance inflammation and cause vascular permeability.

Only a few patients experience persistent inflammation (neutralizing antibodies), while most patients survive the inflammatory responses and clear the virus. The mechanism of antibody-dependent enhancement promotes viral cellular uptake of infectious virus–antibody complexes, and interaction with Fc receptors (FcR), FcR, or other receptors, resulting in enhanced infection of target cells. The interaction of FcR with the virus-anti-S protein-neutralizing antibodies complex facilitates both inflammatory responses and persistent viral replication in the lungs of patients [7].

Peripheral CD4 and CD8 T cells showed reduction and hyperactivation in severe cases. High concentrations of proinflammatory CD4 T cells and cytotoxic granules CD8 T act as antiviral immune responses and overactivation of T cells. Lymphopenia is a critical factor for severity and mortality.

We can observe significantly high blood levels of cytokines and chemokines in patients with COVID-19 infection that included IL1-β, IL1RA, IL7, IL8, IL9, IL10, basic FGF2, GCSF, GMCSF, IFNγ, IP10, MCP1, MIP1α, MIP1β, PDGFB, TNFα, and VEGFA. Severe cases showed high levels of pro-inflammatory cytokines including IL2, IL7, IL10, GCSF, IP10, MCP1, MIP1α, and TNFα [8].

SARS-CoV-2 patients who become critically ill suffer a generalized thrombotic microvascular injury, involving at least the lung and skin, and it appears mediated by intense complement activation, attacking endothelial cell injury and making subsequent activation of the clotting pathway, leading to fibrin deposition. Critical biomarkers consistent with complement-mediated microvascular injury and thrombosis in COVID-19 patients will be important: D-dimers; factor VIII, fibrinogen, and other coagulation factors; antiphospholipid antibodies; C-reactive protein; proinflammatory cytokines, particularly IL-1 and IL-6; circulating complement proteins including C3, C4, C5b-9, and Bb [9].

It is imperative to take into account that not only lung affection is more severe in elderly patients. The occurrence of non-respiratory complications is higher than young people: acute kidney injury, cardiac atrial fibrillation, ventricular fibrillation and clinically significant bradycardia and others [10].

We can correlate the pathophysiology with the main pathologic findings.

In the lungs of pre-symptomatic COVID-19 patients (early phase), we can observe oedema, proteinaceous exudate, and focal hyperplasia of pneumocytes with only patchy inflammatory cellular infiltration, and the absence of hyaline membranes [11].

In fatal cases of COVID-19 pneumonia, the main findings are hyaline membrane formation, fibrin exudates, epithelial damage, and diffuse-type II pneumocyte hyperplasia. In advanced stages, mild thickening of alveolar walls is also evident in some cases. However, mature fibrosis is not observed. With advancing disease, consolidation occurs in severely ill patients, likely due to intra-alveolar organization by fibroblastic proliferation with extracellular matrix formation, and interstitial and thickening. In cases lasting longer than 30 days, interstitial and alveolar fibroblast proliferation, septal thickening, and organizing pneumonia are evident [11].

So the physiopathology of COVID acute respiratory failure is a broad and complex process, where viral, immunological and vascular components coexist. Based on this knowledge, clinicians use a wide variety of empirical treatments: antiviral medical treatment, immunoenhancement therapy, convalescent plasma therapy, auxiliary blood purification treatment, anticoagulants, etc. We need more studies to know which of these treatments are useful or not [12–15].

Future vaccination strategies will need to elicit strong protective antibody responses in older adults, using age-appropriate adjuvants, antiviral and immuno-modulatory treatments [16].

The physiopathology of acute respiratory failure in the elderly affected by COVID-19 is of particular relevance, not only because it is the age group most affected by the disease, and the one with the highest morbidity and mortality, but also because it is the most complex. There is no doubt that we need to progress in our physiopathological knowledge of the elderly, as this will translate into better therapeutic weapons not only for this group but for all patients affected by COVID-19.

References

1. Yuki K, Fujiogi M, Koutsogiannaki S. COVID-19 pathophysiology: a review. Clin Immunol. 2019;215:108427. https://doi.org/10.1016/j.clim.2020.108427.
2. Van den Brand JM, Haagmans BL, Van Riel D, Osterhaus AD, Kuiken T. The pathology and pathogenesis of experimental severe acute respiratory syndrome and influenza in animal models. J Comp Pathol. 2014;151:83–112.
3. Nikhra V. The agent and host factors in COVID-19: exploring pathogenesis and therapeutic implications. Biomed J Sci Tech Res. 2020;27(2):20669–81.
4. Nikolich-Zugich J, Knox KS, Tafich-Rios C, Natt B, Bhattacharya D, Fain MJ. SARS-CoV-2 and COVID-19 in older adults: what we may expect regarding pathogenesis, immune responses, and outcomes. GeroScience. 2020;42:505. https://doi.org/10.1007/s11357-020-00186-0.
5. Poor HD, Ventetuolo CE, Tolbert MD, Chun G, Serrao G, Zeidman A, et al. COVID-19 critical illness pathophysiology driven by diffuse pulmonary thrombi and pulmonary endothelial dysfunction responsive to thrombolysis. Clin Trans Med. 2020; https://doi.org/10.1101/2020.04.17.20057125.
6. Abdulamir A, Hafidh RR. The possible immunological pathways for the variable immuno-pathogenesis of COVID-19 infections among healthy adults, elderly and children. Electron J Gen Med. 2020;17(4):em202. https://doi.org/10.29333/ejgm/7850.
7. Jin Y, Yang H, Ji W, Wu W, Chen S, Zhang W, et al. Virology, epidemiology, pathogenesis, and control of COVID-19. Viruses. 2020;12:372. https://doi.org/10.3390/v12040372.

8. Rothana HA, Byrareddy SN. The epidemiology and pathogenesis of coronavirus disease (COVID-19) outbreak. J Autoimmun. 2020;109:102433. https://doi.org/10.1016/j.jaut.2020.102433.

9. Magro C, Mulvey JJ, Berlin D, Nuovo G, Salvatore S, Harp J, et al. Complement associated microvascular injury and thrombosis in the pathogenesis of severe COVID-19 infection: a report of five cases. Transl Res. 2020;220:1. https://doi.org/10.1016/j.trsl.2020.04.007.

10. Wang L, He W, Yu X, Hu D, Bao M, Liu H, et al. Coronavirus disease 2019 in elderly patients: characteristics and prognostic factors based on 4-week follow-up. J Inf Secur. 2020;80:639–45. https://doi.org/10.1016/j.jinf.2020.03.019.

11. Tian S, Xiong Y, Liu H, Niu L, Gou J, Liao M, et al. Pathological study of the 2019 novel coronavirus disease (COVID-19) through postmortem core biopsies. Mod Pathol. 2020;33:1007. https://doi.org/10.1038/s41379-020-0536-x.

12. Qin C, Zhou L, Hu Z, Zhang S, Yang S, Tao Y, et al. Dysregulation of immune response in patients with coronavirus 2019 (COVID-19) in Wuhan, China. Clin Infect Dis. 2020;2020:ciaa248. https://doi.org/10.1093/cid/ciaa248.

13. Schafer A, Baric R, Ferris MY. Systems approaches to coronavirus pathogenesis. Curr Opin Struct Biol. 2014;6:61–9.

14. Wang L, Wang Y, Ye D, Liu Q. Review of the 2019 novel coronavirus (SARS-CoV-2) based on current evidence. Int J Antimicrob Agents. 2020;55:105948. https://doi.org/10.1016/j.ijantimicag.2020.105948.

15. Kadkhoda K. COVID-19: an Immunopathological view. mSphere. 2020;5:e00344. https://doi.org/10.1128/mSphere.00344-20.

16. Di Gennaro F, Pizzol D, Marotta C, Antunes M, Racalbuto V, Veronese N, et al. Coronavirus diseases (COVID-19) current status and future perspectives: a narrative review. Int J Environ Res Public Health. 2020;17:2690. https://doi.org/10.3390/ijerph17082690.

Escalation Therapy for ARF in Elderly Patient

12

Alejandro Úbeda and Irene Fernández

12.1 Introduction

The prevalence of hypoxic respiratory failure in patients with COVID-19 has been reported in 19%. Recent reports from China showed that 4–13% of COVID-19 patients in these studies received noninvasive positive pressure ventilation (NIPPV), and that 2.3–12% required invasive mechanical ventilation. Although the true incidence of hypoxic respiratory failure in patients with COVID-19 is not clear, it appears that about 14% will develop severe disease requiring oxygen therapy, and 5% will require ICU admission and mechanical ventilation [1]. Some studies have shown that avoiding invasive mechanical ventilation (IMV) significantly decreases the risk of death [2, 3]. This is why choosing an optimal oxygen therapy device is very important for reducing the rates of IMV and mortality while also ensuring patients' safety and comfort [4]. The CDC reported an overall case-fatality rate (CFR) of 2.3%, with a CFR of 14.8% in patients aged 80 years or older [1]. We must consider oxygen therapy if [4, 5]:

Clinical criteria:

- Moderate-severe dyspnea and accessory muscle use or paradoxical abdominal movement.
- Respiratory rate > 30 bpm.

Gasometric criteria:

- $pO_2/FiO_2 < 200$ (or $FiO_2 > 0.4$ to obtain at least 94% SpO_2).
- ARF (pH < 7.35 and $pCO_2 > 45$ mmHg).

A. Úbeda (✉) · I. Fernández
Intensive Care Unit, Hospital Punta de Europa, Algeciras, Spain

N. Vargas, A. M. Esquinas (eds.), *Covid-19 Airway Management and Ventilation Strategy for Critically Ill Older Patients*, https://doi.org/10.1007/978-3-030-55621-1_12

Oxygen delivery systems are generally classified as low-flow or variable-performance devices and high-flow or fixed-performance devices. Low-flow systems provide oxygen at flow rates that are lower than patients' inspiratory demands. When the total ventilation exceeds the capacity of the oxygen reservoir, room air is entrained. The final concentration of oxygen delivered depends on the ventilatory demands of the patient, the size of the oxygen reservoir, and the rate at which the reservoir is filled. At a constant flow, the larger the tidal volume, the lower the FiO_2 and vice versa. In contrast, the high-flow systems provide a constant FiO_2 by delivering the gas at flow rates that exceed the patient's peak inspiratory flow rate and by using devices that entrain a fixed proportion of room air. If the ventilatory demand of the patient is met completely by the system, then it is a high-flow system. In contrast, if the system fails to meet the ventilatory demand of the patient, then it is classified as a low-flow system [4]. There are no randomized or non-randomized studies on the use of oxygen in adults with COVID-19, so recommendations are done using indirect evidence.

12.2   Nasal Cannulae

Nasal cannulae are perhaps the simplest mode of administering low-to-moderate concentrations of inspired oxygen. The short cannulas deliver oxygen directly to the nasopharynx, reducing dead space and inspiratory resistance, and they can deliver a range of oxygen flow rates from 1–6 L/min, corresponding to FiO_2 values of approximately 24–50%. In addition, low-flow oxygen therapy can be continued via nasal cannulas during the administration of air-driven nebulizers for hypercapnic or acidotic patients. In addition, the FiO_2 is affected by a multitude of patient factors, including mouth breathing, degree of nasal congestion, and the respiratory rate (RR). The use of nasal cannulas should therefore target a specific oxygen saturation level which may vary regarding patient's medical history, with ongoing monitoring and titration of the oxygen flow rate to achieve this [6].

12.3   Simple Mask

The Venturi system allows the constant delivery of a fixed concentration of oxygen to the patient. This could be delivered at higher flow rates for tachypneic patients in whom the minute volume might otherwise exceed the available oxygen flow. Each valve is manufactured to deliver only a specific FiO_2, with valves for 24%, 28%, 35%, 40%, and 60% usually available, and a minimum oxygen flow rate, above which the resulting air–oxygen mixture will correspond to the intended ratios. The Venturi system must be used with a face mask and therefore is subject to the usual disadvantages and being more prone to dislodge [6].

12.4 Non-rebreather Mask

A non-rebreather is a mask with a reservoir bag attached and three one-way valves that allow the patient to exhale CO_2 out of the two holes on the mask, but not be able to breathe in air from the room through those ports. By not allowing the patient to breathe in air from the room, which would dilute the concentration of oxygen, this enables the mask deliver close to 100% oxygen, as long as the liter flow is high enough (10–15 L/min of oxygen) [6]. The conventional oxygen therapy to treat hypoxemic patients shows several disadvantages such as the imprecise estimation of the delivered FiO_2, the CO_2-rebreathing with "reservoir" devices, the subject's discomfort due to mask poor tolerance and interference with eating, drinking, speaking, insufficient heating and humidification of the administered oxygen, and the mismatch between the limited amount of the deliverable oxygen flow and the high patient's inspiratory request. Furthermore, conventional oxygen therapy is unable of unloading respiratory muscles and may cause a rise in $PaCO_2$ level leading to the need for mechanical ventilation especially in patients with acute on-chronic hypercapnic respiratory failure. In adults with COVID-19 supplementary oxygen should be started if SpO_2 is <90% and should be maintained no higher than 96% [1].

12.5 High-Flow Oxygen Cannula (HFOC)

HFOC allows us to administer a gas flow of up to 60 L/min using silicone nasal cannulas, with ideal conditions of administered gas temperature and humidity (37 °C and 100% relative humidity). To administrate enough FiO_2, a system capable of administering a high gas flow (from 0 to 60 L/min) and of adjusting the administered FiO_2 is required. As there is less dilution with room air, HFOC can provide enough flow to satisfy the peak inspiratory flow demand of the patient, where the administered FiO_2 comes close to the real value received by the patient. This is because the administered gas flow is not diluted with room air. HFOC also generates a certain positive airway pressure. This is important, since it means that the improvement in oxygenation would be partially due to improved alveolar recruitment, attributable at least in part to the mentioned increase in airway pressure. HFOC also reduces the anatomical dead space and increases alveolar ventilation, decreases respiratory work and increases patient comfort [7]. In an RCT comparing HFNC with NIPPV in patients with acute hypoxic respiratory failure, HFNC resulted in reduced mortality at 90 days (HR, 2.50; 95% CI, 1.31–4.78), but did not significantly affect the need for intubation (50% failure rate in NIPPV vs. 47% in conventional oxygen and 40% in HFNC groups; $p = 0.18$) (71). Another meta-analysis comparing HFNC with NIPPV showed that HFNC reduces the need for intubation of patients, without significantly reducing mortality or ICU length of stay (72). In addition, in SARS, there are reports of increased transmission of disease to healthcare workers, especially nurses, during endotracheal intubation (OR, 6.6; 95% Cl,

2.3–18.9). Although this is a finding based mostly on retrospective observational studies, HFNC does not seem to confer an increased risk of transmission of disease. In studies evaluating bacterial environmental contamination, HFNC presented a contamination risk similar to that of conventional oxygen [1]. Although some authors advised avoiding the use of HFNC in patients with COVID-19 due to the fear of disease transmission, studies supporting this advice are lacking [1]. For adults with COVID-19 and acute hypoxemic ARF despite conventional oxygen therapy, HFNC are recommended over conventional oxygen therapy and noninvasive positive pressure ventilation (NIPPV) [1]. Once physicians realize that conventional oxygen therapy is not enough to properly correct the impaired lung gas exchange and to reduce the burden of respiratory distress, NIPPV becomes the following option whose aim is to avoid the need for IMV. The advantage of NIPPV is to offer the same physiological effects of IMV delivered via endotracheal intubation avoiding its risks, such as ventilator-associated pneumonia, whose incidence rate is higher in the elderly [8]. Three situations could be described [5]: Scenario 1. No medical conditions and hypoxemic respiratory failure. NIPPV is only recommended in selected patients if: (a) $pO_2/FiO_2 > 100$ despite >1 h conventional oxygen. (b) No multiorgan failure (APACHE <20). (c) Endotracheal intubation (ETI) within the next hour if worsen. Scenario 2. Hypoxemic respiratory failure and do-not-intubate (DNI) order. When initiating NIPPV in these patients, we must consider: (a) Target SpO_2 95%. (b) Use high PEEP and low support pressure in order to obtain respiratory tidal volume <9 mL/kg. Scenario 3. Severe COPD exacerbation and hypercapnic acute respiratory failure. Performing a NIV test tolerance may be considered. The use of predictive factors may be useful in the selection-making process even though those with a greater predictive value (clinical-physiological parameters after a trial of NIPPV) are not available before starting ventilation. The finding at baseline of severe acidosis (pH $\leq$ 7.25), remarked "de novo" hypoxemia ($pO_2/FiO_2 \leq 200$ mmHg) and non-pulmonary organ failures are associated with a likelihood of NIV failure. In that scenario we must consider initiating IMV if the patient is eligible for that therapy [9]. The balance between benefit and harm when using NIPPV in adults with COVID-19 is unclear. However, because limited experience with NIPPV in pandemics suggests a high failure rate, any patient receiving NIPPV may be monitored closely and cared for in a setting where intubation can be facilitated in the event of decompensation. Moreover, when resources become stretched, there may be insufficient ability to provide invasive ventilation, and even a moderate chance of success with NIPPV may justify its use [1]. If NIPPV is used, helmet NIPPV has also been shown to reduce exhaled air dispersion and could be an attractive option, if available. A single-center RCT showed decreased intubation and improved mortality from NIPPV delivered by helmet in ARDS patients [10].

12.6 Invasive Mechanical Ventilation (IMV)

While the application of the conservative therapeutic approach based on the solely administration of drugs and oxygen within the context of non-intensive care setting is not dissimilar in the elderly than in adults, the choice of administering mechanical ventilation in ICU in octogenarians is controversial. In fact, despite the prognosis of patients undergoing mechanical ventilation has not been shown to be different in the elderly than in the younger population, the former usually receive less intensive and expensive care than the latter having the same degree of clinical-physiological derangement. This is particularly evident in the elderly with chronic cardiopulmonary diseases hospitalized for an episode of ARF for whom the denial of ICU admission is often determined by an unjustified pessimistic prognostic perspective shown by physicians. Even if the "age-based" restriction access to higher level of care is not justified by the existing data, in some institutions the label of DNI order may be applied to octogenarians with chronic advanced respiratory disease [11]. IMV should be considered for patients with ARDS, particularly those with moderate or severe ARDS ($PaO_2/FiO_2 \leq 200$ mmHg). A ventilatory strategy recommended is the one that prioritizes low-tidal volumes (TV) and low plateau pressures, so-called "lung-protective ventilation." The TV should be decreased over several hours to a goal of 6 mL/kg IBW. Also should be decreased further if necessary to achieve a plateau pressure [9].

12.7 Extracorporeal Membrane Oxygenation (ECMO)

The Society of Critical Care Medicine recommend VV ECMO in the management of ARDS in those in whom refractory hypoxemia persist despite optimized ventilation, the use of rescue therapies (such as the use of inhaled pulmonary vasodilators) and proning. They provide an algorithm to help guide decision-making with the following criteria promoting a recommendation for early ECMO usage:

- $paO_2:FiO_2 < 80$ mmHg for >6 h.
- $paO_2:FiO_2 < 50$ mmHg for >3 h.
- pH < 7.25 with $PaCO_2 \geq 60$ mmHg for >6 h.

In the current pandemic and wave of new COVID-19 cases, ECMO should be considered only in those with a good prognosis; those without significant comorbidities, less than 7 days on mechanical ventilation and should not be considered in the critically ill elderly due to poor outcomes regardless of ECMO support [1].

References

1. Alhazzani W, Moller MH, Arabi YM, et al. Surviving sepsis campaign: guidelines on the management of critically ill adults with coronavirus disease 2019 (COVID-19). Crit Care Med. 2020;48:e440.
2. Azevedo LC, Caruso P, Silva UV, et al. Outcomes for patients with cancer admitted to the ICU requiring ventilatory support: results from a prospective multicenter study. Chest. 2014;146(2):257–66.
3. Azoulay E, Mokart D, Pène F, et al. Outcomes of critically ill patients with hematologic malignancies: prospective multicenter data from France and Belgium—a Groupe de Recherche Respiratoire en reanimation Onco-Hématologique study. J Clin Oncol. 2013;31(22):2810–8.

4. Zhu Y, Yin H, Zhang R, et al. High-flow nasal cannula oxygen therapy versus conventional oxygen therapy in patients with acute respiratory failure: a systematic review and meta-analysis of randomized controlled trials. BMC Pulm Med. 2017;17:201.
5. Cinesi C, Peñuelas O, Luján MI, et al. Recomendaciones de consenso respecto al soporte respiratorio no invasivo en el paciente adulto con insuficiencia respiratoria aguda secundaria a infección por SARS-CoV-2. Med Int. 2020; https://doi.org/10.1016/j.medin.2020.03.005.
6. Brill S, Wedzicha J. Oxygen therapy in acute exacerbations of chronic obstructive pulmonary disease. Int J COPD. 2014;9:1241–52.
7. Masclans JR, Pérez-Terán P, Roca O. The role of high-flow oxygen therapy in acute respiratory failure. Med Int. 2015;39(8):505–15.
8. Frat JP, Thille AW, Mercat A, et al. High-flow oxygen through nasal cannula in acute hypoxemic respiratory failure. N Engl J Med. 2015;372:2185–96.
9. Walter J, Corbridge T, Singer B. Invasive mechanical ventilation. South Med J. 2018 December;111(12):746–53.
10. Patel BK, Wolfe KS, Pohlman AS, Hall JB, Kress JP. Effect of noninvasive ventilation delivered by helmet vs face mask on the rate of endotracheal intubation in patients with acute respiratory distress syndrome: a randomized clinical trial. JAMA. 2016;315:2435–41.
11. Scala R. Challenges on non-invasive ventilation to treat acute respiratory failure in the elderly. BMC Pulm Med. 2016;16:150.

Oxygen Therapy: Liberal Versus Conservative in Older Patients with COVID Disease

13

Loredana Tibullo, Nicola Vargas, and Antonio M. Esquinas

13.1 Introduction

The management of acute respiratory failure is more complicated in elderly patients. The reasons behind this difficulty are mainly related to the frailty and the comorbidities. In particular, the frailty is characterised by a decline in physiological capacity across several organ systems, with a resultant increased susceptibility to stressors. In a few words, frailty means diminished organ reserve, including that of the lung. The first step in the management of acute respiratory failure remains to treat hypoxemia with oxygen therapy. The primary rationale of oxygen (O_2) therapy is to prevent and correct arterial hypoxaemia (reduction of O_2 in the blood) and any resulting hypoxia (the decrease of the O_2 in the tissues) in patients with or at risk for impaired pulmonary gas exchange. The hypoxaemia is characterised by the partial pressure of O_2 less than 60 mmHg in blood gas analysis or a SaO_2 of <90% while breathing in room air [1]. Besides, over the last years, most acute treatment algorithms recommended the liberal use of a high fraction of inspired oxygen, even without first confirming the presence of a hypoxic insult. For example, for more than a century, supplemental oxygen has been used routinely in the treatment of patients with suspected acute myocardial infarction. The use of additional oxygen therapy in acute coronary syndromes (ACS) and cardiac emergencies has demonstrated to be controversial. In 2010, the American Heart Association (AHA) stated that oxygen should be delivered to patients with breathlessness, signs of heart failure, shock, or an

L. Tibullo (✉)
Medicine Department, Ward of Internal Medicine, San Giuseppe Moscati Hospital, Aversa, Italy

N. Vargas
Geriatric and Intensive Geriatric Cares, San Giuseppe Moscati Hospital, Avellino, Italy

A. M. Esquinas
Intensive Care Unit, Hospital Morales Meseguer, Murcia, Spain

© The Editor(s) (if applicable) and The Author(s), under exclusive license to
Springer Nature Switzerland AG 2020
N. Vargas, A. M. Esquinas (eds.), *Covid-19 Airway Management and Ventilation Strategy for Critically Ill Older Patients*, https://doi.org/10.1007/978-3-030-55621-1_13

arterial oxyhaemoglobin saturation <94% (Class I, LOE C) and not to all patients with ACS. Non-invasive monitoring of blood oxygen saturation can be useful to decide on the need for oxygen administration [2]. In 2015, some data questioned the consolidated clinical use of supplemental oxygen therapy. The Australian Air Versus Oxygen in Myocardial Infarction (AVOID) trial supported an adverse effect of oxygen. The trial reported larger infarct sizes in patients with ST-segment elevation myocardial infarction (STEMI) who received oxygen than in those who did not receive oxygen [3]. The history of oxygen supplementation in ACS is an example of the binary therapeutic option (liberal versus conservative use of oxygen). A Cochrane report from 2016 did not show any evidence supporting the routine use of oxygen in the treatment of patients with myocardial infarction [4]. In the same way for the treatment of stroke, the guidelines have affirmed that oxygen therapy may be harmful if used for non-hypoxemic patients with mild-moderate strokes [5]. Starting from these examples in this chapter, the authors analysed the evidence of oxygen therapy in the treatment of acute critical patients and acute respiratory distress syndrome (ARDS). The authors will investigate the use of oxygen therapy in light of the available physiopathological patterns of acute respiratory failure of COVID-19 disease.

13.2   Oxygen Therapy in Critical Conditions

The administration of supplemental oxygen is a cornerstone of care in the intensive care unit (ICU). Moreover, the data of many randomised controlled trials (RCTs) comparing liberal versus conservative oxygen for various critical conditions are not conclusive [6]. In one sizeable single-centre RCT among 480 ICU patients, subjects were randomised either into conservative oxygen supplementation (PaO_2 70–100 mmHg or oxygen saturations 94–98%) or into conventional oxygen supplementation (PaO_2 100–150 mmHg or oxygen saturations 97–100%). Among critically ill patients with an ICU length of stay of 72 h or longer, a conservative protocol for oxygen therapy vs. conventional therapy resulted in lower ICU mortality. Furthermore, the preliminary data were based on unplanned early termination of the trial [7]. Starting from the recommendation that the ARDS requires to reach a partial target pressure of arterial oxygen (PaO_2) between 55 and 80 mmHg, Barrot et al. showed that among patients with ARDS, early exposure to a conservative-oxygenation strategy with a PaO_2 between 55 and 70 mmHg did not increase survival at 28 days [8]. A multicentric investigation considered patients who are undergoing mechanical ventilation in ICU. The authors randomly assigned 1000 adult patients who require mechanical ventilation in the ICU to receive conservative or conventional oxygen therapy. In the two groups, the default lower limit for oxygen saturation as measured by pulse oximetry (SpO_2) was 90%. In the conservative group, oxygen therapy aimed to maintain SpO_2 at >90% and <97%. In the control group, the liberal oxygen therapy provided that no upper limit to SpO_2 with a targeted lower limit of >90%. The use of $FiO_2 < 30\%$ was discouraged. The primary outcome was the number of ventilator-free days from randomisation until day 28.

The study showed that the number of ventilator-free days did not differ significantly between the conservative-oxygen group and the usual-oxygen group [9]. Nevertheless, the best practices for ARDS suggested over last years the use of low tidal volume strategy, PEEP titration, avoidance of hyperoxia, and a conservative fluid strategy. The rationale of the conservative use of oxygen is that it may eliminate hyperoxaemia, reduce oxygen exposure, diminish lung and systemic oxidative injury, and thereby increase the number of ventilator-free days (days alive and free from mechanical ventilation. Excessive oxygen supplementation may have detrimental pulmonary and systemic effects because of enhanced oxidative stress and inflammation. Hyperoxia-induced lung injury includes altered surfactant protein composition, reduced mucociliary clearance and histological damage, resulting in atelectasis, decreased lung compliance and increased risk of infections. Also, it causes vasoconstriction, reduction in coronary blood flow and cardiac output and may alter microvascular perfusion [10]. Hyperoxia leads to higher mortality in critically ill patients, especially in patients with cardiac arrest and extracorporeal life support (ELS) [11].

13.3   Oxygen Therapy in COVID-19 Disease

The WHO clinical management of severe acute respiratory infection (SARI) when COVID-19 disease is suspected recommended to provide supplemental oxygen therapy immediately to patients with SARI and respiratory distress, hypoxaemia or shock and target $SpO_2 > 94\%$. The WHO recommendations remarked that adults with emergency signs (obstructed or absent breathing, severe respiratory distress, central cyanosis, shock, coma, or convulsions) should receive airway management and oxygen therapy during resuscitation to target $SpO_2 \geq 94\%$. Oxygen therapy should be initiated at 5 L/min and titrate flow rates to reach goal $SpO_2 \geq 93\%$ during resuscitation, or use a face mask with reservoir bag (at 10–15 L/min) if the patient in critical condition. Once the patient is stable, the target is $>90\%$ SpO_2 [12]. Furthermore, patients may continue to have increased work of breathing or hypoxemia even when oxygen is delivered via a face mask with reservoir bag (flow rates of 10–15 L/min, which is typically the minimum flow required to maintain bag inflation). Hence, the hypoxemic respiratory failure may lead to the ARDS that commonly results from an intrapulmonary ventilation-perfusion mismatch [13]. Some authors advised that the patients with COVID-19 pneumonia, satisfying the Berlin criteria of ARDS, present an atypical form of the syndrome. They noted that the primary characteristics observed were the dissociation between the relatively well-preserved lung mechanics and the severity of hypoxemia [14]. The authors identified the development of a time-related COVID disease spectrum within two "phenotypes": *Type L* (characterised by Low elastance (i.e. high compliance), Low ventilation-to-perfusion ratio, Low lung weight and Low recruitability) and *Type H* (characterised by High elastance, High right-to-left shunt, High lung weight and High recruitability). The first step to treat the Type L is to reverse hypoxemia with liberal oxygen therapy. If the patient is not yet breathless, it is possible to increase the FiO_2 and improve the outcome. Besides in Type L patients with dyspnoea, several non-invasive options are available: high-flow nasal cannula (HFNC), continuous positive airway pressure (CPAP) or non-invasive ventilation (NIV). Type H patients as severe ARDS require higher PEEP, if compatible with haemodynamics, prone positioning and extracorporeal support [15].

Many questions remain still open on COVID-19 disease. Many authors suggest studying the impact of hyperoxaemia in damaging alveolar epithelial cells. These effects may be evident using nasal flow oxygen in the lung during COVID-19 disease. But, the autopsy findings and the referred scientific literature will help to clarify the pathogenesis and indicate the most accurate oxygen treatment.

13.4 Conclusion

The binary therapeutic option (liberal versus conservative use of oxygen studied over the last years) during the actual pandemic in which severe hypoxemic state characterise the COVID disease need a possible ad hoc RCT. But, the administration of oxygen to relief the severe hypoxemia even with a liberal way of delivery is acceptable. This first step is crucial to evaluate further non-invasive and invasive therapeutic options.

References

1. Kallstrom TJ. American Association for Respiratory Care (AARC) AARC clinical practice guideline: oxygen therapy for adults in the acute care facility—2002 revision & update. Respir Care. 2002;47(6):717–20.
2. O'Connor RE, Brady W, Brooks SC, et al. Part 10: acute coronary syndromes: 2010 American Heart Association guidelines for cardiopulmonary resuscitation and emergency cardiovascular care. Circulation. 2010;122(18 Suppl 3):S787–817. https://doi.org/10.1161/CIRCULATIONAHA.110.971028.
3. Stub D, Smith K, Bernard S, Nehme Z, Michael Stephenson RN, Bray JE, Cameron P, Barger B, Ellims AH, Taylor AJ, Meredith IT, Kaye DM, on behalf of the AVOID Investigators. Air versus oxygen in ST-segment–elevation myocardial infarction. Circulation. 2015;131:2143–50.
4. Cabello JB, Burls A, Emparanza JI, Bayliss SE, Quinn T. Oxygen therapy for acute myocardial infarction. Cochrane Database Syst Rev. 2016;12:CD007160.
5. O'Driscoll BR, et al. BTS guidelines 2017. Thorax. 2017;72:i1–i90. https://doi.org/10.1136/thoraxjnl-2016-209729.
6. Vargas M, Servillo G. Liberal versus conservative oxygen therapy in critically ill patients: using the fragility index to determine robust results. Crit Care. 2019;23:132. https://doi.org/10.1186/s13054-018-2165-z.
7. Girardis M, Busani S, Damiani E, et al. Effect of conservative vs conventional oxygen therapy on mortality among patients in an intensive care unit: the Oxygen-ICU randomized clinical trial. JAMA. 2016;316(15):1583–9. https://doi.org/10.1001/jama.2016.11993.
8. Barrot L, Asfar P, Mauny F, Winiszewski H, Montini F, Badie J, Quenot J-P, Pili-Floury S, Bouhemad B, Louis G, Souweine B, Collange O, Pottecher J, Levy B, Puyraveau M, Vettoretti L, Constantin J-M, Capellier G. Liberal or conservative oxygen therapy for acute respiratory distress syndrome. N Engl J Med. 2020;382(11):999–1008. https://doi.org/10.1056/NEJMoa1916431.

9. The ICU-ROX Investigators and the Australian and new Zealand Intensive Care Society Clinical Trials Group. Conservative oxygen therapy during mechanical ventilation in the ICU. N Engl J Med. 2020;382:989–98. https://doi.org/10.1056/NEJMoa1903297.
10. Damiani E, Donati A, Girardis M. Oxygen in the critically ill: friend or foe? Curr Opin Anaesthesiol. 2018;31(2):129–35.
11. Ni YN, Wang YM, Liang BM, Liang ZA. The effect of hyperoxia on mortality in critically ill patients: a systematic review and meta analysis. BMC Pulm Med. 2019;19(1):53. https://doi.org/10.1186/s12890-019-0810-1.
12. WHO. Oxygen therapy for children: a manual for health workers. Geneva: World Health Organization; 2013. http://www.who.int/maternal_child_adolescent/documents/child-oxygen-therapy/en/. Accessed 10 March 2020.
13. Rhodes A, Evans LE, Alhazzani W, Levy MM, Antonelli M, Ferrer R, et al. Surviving Sepsis campaign: international guidelines for Management of Sepsis and Septic Shock: 2016. Intensive Care Med. 2017;43(3):304–77. https://doi.org/10.1007/s00134-017-4683-6.
14. Gattinoni L, Coppola S, Cressoni M, Busana M, Rossi S, Chiumello D. Covid-19 does not lead to a "typical" acute respiratory distress syndrome. Am J Respir Crit Care Med. 2020;201(10):1299–300. https://doi.org/10.1164/rccm.202003-0817LE.
15. Gattinoni L, Chiumello D, Caironi P, et al. COVID-19 pneumonia: different respiratory treatments for different phenotypes? Intensive Care Med. 2020;46:1099. https://doi.org/10.1007/s00134-020-06033-2.

The Role of Non-invasive Ventilation

14

Hadeer S. Harb, Yasmin M. Madney,
Mohamed E. Abdelrahim, and Haitham Saeed

14.1 Introduction

Patients with severe COVID-19 usually develop acute respiratory distress syndrome (ARDS) characterised by acute hypoxemic respiratory failure (HRF) and bilateral pulmonary infiltrates [1, 2]. The common reason for HRF occurring in the course of ARDS is the ventilation-perfusion mismatch or the intrapulmonary shunt [3]. Generally, HRF is defined as an acute condition where the arterial oxygen tension is below 60 mmHg on room air or oxygen is required to maintain measurements of pulse oximetry above 90% with low or normal partial carbon dioxide pressure [4]. Therapeutic options are limited to target the ongoing pathological processes of ARDS, and hence mechanical ventilation continues to be the mainstay for patient management [5]. Non-invasive ventilation (NIV) and high flow nasal cannula oxygen therapy (HFNC) can play a role in providing respiratory support to COVID-19 patients before developing severe HRF or in circumstances where there is limited access to more invasive techniques [1].

14.2 Indications of Non-invasive Ventilation (Table 14.1)

Indications for NIV include mild respiratory failure where partial oxygen pressure (PaO_2)/fraction of inspired oxygen (FiO_2) equal to 200–300 or new conditions of moderate respiratory failure where PaO_2/FiO_2 equivalent to 150–200 and the work of breathing is not high [6]. Airway management will significantly decrease disease complications and improve rehabilitation [7]. The patient should be closely monitored for 1–2 h after receiving HFNC or NIV to assess the success of therapy. If the

H. S. Harb · Y. M. Madney · M. E. Abdelrahim (✉) · H. Saeed
Clinical Pharmacy Department, Faculty of Pharmacy, Beni-suef University, Beni-suef, Egypt

© The Editor(s) (if applicable) and The Author(s), under exclusive license to
Springer Nature Switzerland AG 2020
N. Vargas, A. M. Esquinas (eds.), *Covid-19 Airway Management and Ventilation Strategy for Critically Ill Older Patients*, https://doi.org/10.1007/978-3-030-55621-1_14

Table 14.1 NIV indications in respiratory failure—COVID-19

Mild ARDS	$PaO_2/FiO_2 = 200–300$
Moderate ARDS	$PaO_2/FiO_2 = 150–200$ and the work of breathing is not high
Older patients with severe ARDS	After a multidimensional evaluation if palliative or end-of-life context; If ICU beds not sufficient; close monitoring is required

patient's condition is not improved or even worsened, then invasive ventilation must be considered [8]. Early intubation must be considered in patients with severe hypoxia or those who exhibit respiratory/cardiac arrest to avoid the prolonged application of HFNC or NIV and the additional risk to which the medical staff is exposed due to the continued usage [9]. The management of ARF with NIV is a primary mean to treat older patients in the presence of negative expected outcome in ICU (as a palliative measure) or reduced resources and with reduced availability of beds. Close monitoring is necessary.

14.3 Technique

Mostly, NIV is delivered by two techniques, either positive pressure or negative pressure where the positive pressure manoeuvre directly inflates the lungs by the applied pressure. In a negative pressure technique, the air is drawn into the lungs via the upper airway under the effect of the pressure externally applied to the thorax and the abdomen. The most commonly referred technique is non-invasive positive pressure ventilation (NPPV) in supporting acute patients, and it is of two forms: continuous positive airway pressure (CPAP) and bi-level positive airway pressure (BiPAP) [10]. Additionally, HFNC is increasingly applied as a therapeutic modality for HRF management, where a heated and humidified gas is supplied in higher flow rates than conventional oxygen delivery systems [11, 12]. Clinical benefits associated with HFNC use in HRF patients include decreasing respiratory effort, increasing oxygenation and improving dynamic compliance [12]. Approximately 11% of severe COVID-19 patients used HFNC in Wuhan during this pandemic, but administering higher flow rates is associated with elevated virus aerosolisation [13]. Some authors suggest that some procedures capable of generating aerosols have been associated with increased risk of SARS transmission such as NIV. However, the most consistent risk is related to tracheal intubation [14]. However, human laboratory data suggest that NIV does not generate aerosols, but this aspect will be investigated in the chapter "the problem of aerosolization".

14.4 Conclusion

NIV and HFNC can provide means of respiratory support in COVID-19 patients experiencing mild or moderate respiratory failure with the need of close monitoring to early determine the failure of such techniques. In this situation, other alternative invasive options may be considered. Virus aerosolisation is the major limitation of NIV use in COVID-19 patients which necessitates specific safety measures to be taken.

References

1. Murthy S, Gomersall CD, Fowler RA. Care for critically ill patients with COVID-19. JAMA. 2020;323:1499.
2. Yang X, et al. Clinical course and outcomes of critically ill patients with SARS-CoV-2 pneumonia in Wuhan, China: a single-centered, retrospective, observational study. Lancet Respir Med. 2020;8:P475–81.
3. World Health Organization. Clinical management of severe acute respiratory infection when Middle East respiratory syndrome coronavirus (MERS-CoV) infection is suspected: interim guidance. Geneva: World Health Organization; 2019.
4. Hukins C, Murphy M, Edwards T. Dose–response characteristics of noninvasive ventilation in acute respiratory failure. ERJ Open Res. 2020;6(1):00041-2019.
5. Fan E, et al. An official American Thoracic Society/European Society of Intensive Care Medicine/Society of Critical Care Medicine clinical practice guideline: mechanical ventilation in adult patients with acute respiratory distress syndrome. Am J Respir Crit Care Med. 2017;195(9):1253–63.
6. Marraro GA, Spada C. Consideration of the respiratory support strategy of severe acute respiratory failure caused by SARS-CoV-2 infection in children. Zhongguo Dang Dai Er Ke Za Zhi. 2020;22(3):183–94.
7. Airway management of COVID-19. patients with severe pneumonia. Zhonghua Er Bi Yan Hou Tou Jing Wai Ke Za Zhi. 2020;55(4):E001.
8. Cascella M, et al. Features, evaluation and treatment coronavirus (COVID-19), in Stat Pearls. Treasure Island, FL: Stat Pearls Publishing Stat Pearls Publishing LLC; 2020.
9. Brewster DJ, et al. Consensus statement: safe airway society principles of airway management and tracheal intubation specific to the COVID-19 adult patient group. Med J Aust. 2020;212(10):1.
10. Scala R, Pisani L. Noninvasive ventilation in acute respiratory failure: which recipe for success? Eur Respir Rev. 2018;27(149):180029.
11. Madney YM, et al. The influence of changing interfaces on aerosol delivery within high flow oxygen setting in adults: an in-vitro study. J Drug Deliv Sci Technol. 2020;55:101365.
12. Hui DS, et al. Exhaled air dispersion during high-flow nasal cannula therapy versus CPAP via different masks. Eur Respir J. 2019;53(4):1802339.
13. Lucchini A, et al. The "helmet bundle" in COVID-19 patients undergoing non invasive ventilation. Intensive Crit Care Nurs. 2020;58:102859.
14. Tran K, Cimon K, Severn M, Pessoa-Silva CL, Conly J. Aerosol generating procedures and risk of transmission of acute respiratory infections to healthcare workers: a systematic review. PLoS One. 2012;7(4):e35797. https://doi.org/10.1371/journal.pone.0035797.

The Invasive Ventilation in Older Patients: The Timing

15

U. T. K. U. Tughan

Coronavirus disease 2019 (COVID-19) is the third coronavirus infection after severe acute respiratory syndrome (SARS) and Middle East respiratory syndrome (MERS). The number of people diagnosed with COVID-19 worldwide crossed the 3.5 million and deaths crossed 245 thousand on May 3, 2020; the case fatality rate across 215 countries and territories was 6.9% [1, 2].

Although Coronavirus disease (COVID-19), which was first described in Wuhan, China, in mid-December 2019, was considered as a severe acute respiratory infection (SARI) [3], in the later stages of the pandemic it turned out that SARI is the most important but not the only problem. Beyond just being a simple viral pneumonia, it was understood to be a complex process that manifests itself with manifestations of ARF, ARDS, shock, thromboembolic event, multiple organ failure. The best evidence that COVID-19 is a complex multisystem clinical syndrome, not simply a simple viral pneumonia, is that patients required basic and advanced cardiac support, kidney, neurological and hepatic support as well as respiratory support [4–7].

The multisystem manifestation of a COVID-19 infection is caused by a combination of specific host-defense responses with associated inflammatory activity and microvascular involvement with pronounced coagulopathy and a strong inclination to develop thromboembolic complications. Patients who had cytokine storm are at highest risk of multisystem failure and thus significant mortality. The hyperinflammatory tissue response leads to drastic multiple organ dysfunction affecting almost all of systems consisting of lungs, heart, kidneys, nerves, muscles, gastrointestinal tract, and brain. SARS-CoV-2 virus have the capability to infect endothelial cells (endotheliitis) via the ACE2 receptors, with release of cytokines. This process makes them more adhesive and increased coagulation. Patients with COVID-19

U. T. K. U. Tughan (✉)
Department of Anaesthesiology and Reanimation, General Intensive Care Unit, Yeditepe University Medical Faculty, Istanbul, Turkey

may present the following clinical patterns; - hypercoagulability with high levels of D-dim, - fibrinogen and factor VIII; - venous thromboembolism; - vascular inflammation and in the presence of this condition large proximal pulmonary artery thrombi or micro-thrombi. The autoptic results, performed in patients with COVID-19, reported hemorrhage and small thrombi areas as well as findings related to DAD (diffuse alveolar damage) [8–11].

In addition to the variety and duration of treatment for this complex and dynamic process, aggressive treatments after instant determinations of natural pathology of disease suggest that patients are susceptible to a serious potential iatrogenic effect.

Although these severely hypoxemic patients share the same etiology (SARS-CoV-2) and fill most of the conditions by definition of Berlin ARDS, they can be quite different from each other, the same disease actually offers an impressive non-uniformity. Albeit the common denominator is severe hypoxemia, the findings vary from silent hypoxemia with normal breathing to pronounced dyspnea, from deep hypocapnia to hypercapnia, from those who respond to high pressures or benefit from prone position to those who do not.

Because of these nonstandard clinical courses, there are hypotheses suggested by the authors to explain the pathophysiology of respiratory failure in COVID-19 cases. As Ottestad et al. underline, the common clinical pattern is the marked mismatch between the severely impaired gas exchange despite the relatively well-preserved lung compliance. This is manifested by fewer signs of respiratory distress, incompatible with the severity of hypoxemia (silent hypoxia) [12].

Respiratory failure in COVID-19 can be classified, considering that the alveolar arterial oxygen difference (delta $P_{(A-a)}O_2$) would be more useful in evaluating the pathophysiological background of hypoxemia. Hypoxemia associated with normal alveolar arterial O_2 difference and high pCO_2 suggests hypoventilation. Hypoxemia with increased alveolar arterial O_2 difference suggests ventilation perfusion mismatch or intrapulmonary shunt. The improvement of hypoxemia with external oxygen is seen in V/P mismatch, while PO_2 does not improve in intrapulmonary shunt [13].

After the mechanical ventilation decision is taken, the primary issue should be not to cause additional damage due to the treatment to be performed. Because mechanical ventilation alone does not cure the patient, on the contrary, it mostly just keeps patients alive until their own biological mechanisms are able to circumvent the coronavirus [13]. Due to the abovementioned basic concern, it may be a solution not to intubate unless absolutely necessary to prevent secondary damage due to the ventilator. Gattinoni et al. in a same manner expressed that all to be done is "buying time" with minimal additional damage when ventilating patients [14].

Based on detailed evaluation of the COVID-19 patient's clinical courses, authors [15] hypothesize that the different COVID-19 patterns found at presentation in the emergency department depend on the interaction between three factors:

1. The severity of the infection, the host response, physiological reserve, and comorbidities.
2. The ventilatory responsiveness of the patient to hypoxemia.

3. The time elapsed between the onset of the disease and the observation in the hospital.

In the article [15], it was stated that after the interaction of these factors, the disease manifested with different phenotypes:

- **Type L**
  - Characterized by
    Low elastance (*or high compliance*)
    Low ventilation to perfusion ratio
    Low lung weight
    Low recruitability
- **Type H**
  - Characterized by
    High elastance
    High right-to-left shunt
    High lung weight
    High recruitability

When published COVID-19 case presentations are analyzed, it is seen that even if mortality rates differ due to inequality in the distribution of the number of patients who are still in bed, a significant group of patients are elderly and have high comorbidity [6, 16]. In the analysis of hospitalized patients with COVID-19 in New York City, 14.2% of patients were treated at ICU, 12.2% of them received invasive mechanical ventilation, 21% of patients died in total, and the mortality rate of patients who underwent mechanical ventilation was 88.1% [16]. Patients who died in ICU (81.3% 0–43.4%) and received invasive mechanical ventilation rates (79.9% – 41.8%) were higher in the 18–65 age group compared to group of older than 65 years age [16]. In the same study, patients with hypertension among the died patients were reported to be less likely to be cared for in the intensive care unit and to receive invasive mechanical ventilation than those without hypertension [16]. In another study, it has been reported that multivariable regression showed increasing odds of in-hospital death associated with older age (odds ratio 1.10, 95% CI 1.03–1.17, per year increase; $p = 0.0043$) [6]. The mortality rate in patients who require invasive mechanical ventilation is high. The median time from illness onset to invasive mechanical ventilation was 14.5 days and ventilator-associated pneumonia occurred in 31% of patients requiring invasive mechanical ventilation [6].

26% of patients necessitate admission to ICU because of the onset of acute respiratory distress syndrome. Patients treated in the ICU, compared with patients not treated in the ICU, were older (median age, 66 years vs. 51 years) and were more likely to have underlying comorbidities (72.2% vs. 37.3%). About 11.1% cases received high-flow oxygen therapy, 41.7% received noninvasive ventilation, and 47.2% received invasive ventilation in the ICU [4].

It has been reported that the earliest extubation occurred 8 days after initiation of invasive mechanical ventilation, which suggests that acute respiratory failure due to

COVID-19 may require prolonged mechanical ventilation and that readiness for extubation is unlikely to occur early in patients receiving mechanical ventilation. Of patients who were extubated, the age range was 23–88 years, which suggests that age may not be the sole indicator for successful extubation [5]. It was reported that 13% of the patients received noninvasive and 4% received invasive mechanical ventilation. Noninvasive mechanical ventilation was performed between 4 and 22 days (median 9 days [IQR 7–19]) while invasive mechanical ventilation was performed for 3–20 days (median 17 [12–19]). P-SIMV mode is mostly used, oxygen concentration is applied between 35 and 100%, and PEEP is reported to be used between 6 and 12 cm H_2O [17].

In a study in which data of 1591 cases were shared [7], it is reported that 99% of the patients taken to the ICU received mechanical ventilation, 88% of them were treated with endotracheal intubation and mechanical ventilation, and 11% were treated with noninvasive ventilation. While invasive mechanical ventilation is used in 88% of young patients, it is reported to be used in 89% of elderly patients. This distribution is between 11% and 10% for noninvasive ventilation. Unlike previous reports, noninvasive ventilation is reported to be used more frequently in the intensive care unit and outside [7]. Although a high rate of high-flow nasal cannula (HFNC) and noninvasive ventilation (NIV) is used in patients, it is uncertain whether "delayed intubation" has adversely affected the results of some patients [18].

A prospective observational cohort study that investigated the clinical features and predictor risk factors for mortality of elderly patients reported that 35% of patients admitted to the ICU received mechanical ventilation treatment [19]. While a significant difference in age-related morbidity was observed, it was reported that elderly patients tend to stay in shorter hospitals and were associated with a low survival. There was no significant difference between age groups in terms of length of hospital stay before being admitted to the intensive care unit. In the elderly group of patients, multivariate analysis related to hospital mortality is reported as comorbid diseases, presence of infection, infections acquired in the ICU, organ dysfunctions rather than mechanical ventilation application as a significant variable. The most important independent variables: the impaired level of consciousness (OR: 2.279, 95% CI = 1.207–4.304, $P = 0.011$), infection on admission (2.114, 95% CI = 1.269–3.520, $P = 0.004$), and ICU-acquired infection (1.977, 95% CI = 1.085–3.601, $P = 0.026$) were reported [19]. On the other hand, Esteban et al. reported that variables associated with mortality of elderly patients receiving mechanical ventilation were acute renal failure and shock [20]. In another study, the factors correlated with increased hospital mortality of elderly ICU patients were acute respiratory failure, use of mechanical ventilation, and inotropes [21].

In the study aiming to determine the relationship between age and in-hospital mortality of elderly patients admitted to the intensive care unit, who needed and did not require invasive ventilation support, age was strongly correlated with mortality in the subgroup of invasively ventilated patients, and multivariate adjusted rates increased with increasing age (OR = 1.60, 95% CI = 1.01–2.54 for 65–74 years old and OR = 2.68, 95% CI = 1.58–4.56 for ≥75 years). As a result of the study, it was reported that the combination of advanced age and invasive mechanical ventilation is strongly associated with in-hospital mortality [22]. In patients treated with invasive mechanical ventilation in intensive care, age is an independent determinant in increasing mortality, but precise quantitative description of the aforementioned change has not been made [22]. The association of age and invasive mechanical ventilation is closely related to mortality [23]. These results may provide additional evidence for the development of new and special invasive mechanical ventilation strategies or the liberal indication of noninvasive mechanical ventilation for elderly patients admitted to the intensive care unit for acute respiratory failure [22].

In the study, the purpose of which was to evaluate the survival rates and functional status of elderly mechanical ventilation patients, survival rates, after hospitalization and 3, 6, and 12 months later, it was found to be 33%, 28%, 25%, and 22%, respectively [24]. As a result of the study, it was reported that in elderly patients treated with mechanical ventilation, the results immediately after ventilation and in the long term are poor, and in this group of patients, a comprehensive assessment of the results of the treatment with mechanical ventilation is required to provide reliable information to patients, families, practitioners, and the community on which life or death decisions can be based [23].

Management of acute respiratory failure in the elderly should be planned not only with the technical aspects of the ventilator and non-ventilator related strategies, but also by taking into account the ethical and economic issues [25]. This entire approach should be planned taking into account the nature of the disease, the level of patient awareness, achieving shared goals, health resources, and the team's expertise in ventilation and intensive care therapy [26]. Although the use of NIV and HFNO remains a good option for the elderly, it is vital for the physician to determine the correct and appropriate selection, appropriate settings and timing based on the case. This choice is also related to the EOL status and attitude in increasing the level of treatment, especially in elderly patients [24]. The use of NIV has markedly increased over the past few years. Persons of advanced age and patients with multiple comorbidities were associated with more frequent NIV use [27].

Although mortality rates are higher both in ICU and in hospital for elderly patients, this does not mean that resources comparatively increased due to mechanical ventilation time, incidence of re-intubation or tracheotomy. Elderly patients with similar mechanical ventilation times have higher mortality than younger patients. It is reported that this difference is associated with higher rates of pneumonia, sepsis, and trauma [28, 29]. The elderly patients who received mechanical ventilation had increased disability compared to those who did not, based on the previous functional status [30].

In subjects with ARDS, the results in the subgroup analysis indicated a higher mortality in the elderly subject group [31–35]. In a study evaluating the clinical features of COVID-19 patients according to their age distribution, the rate of ARDS was higher in elderly patients (22.22% vs. 5.26%), and while NIV administration rates did not show a significant difference compared to age groups (5.56% vs. 5.26%), invasive MV rates were reported to be significantly higher in the elderly (22.22% vs. 7.89%) [36].

In RCT study examining the effects of respiratory rehabilitation (RR) on respiratory functions in elderly patients with COVID-19 disease who was discharged from the hospital with the positive results, improvement in respiratory functions, quality of life, and anxiety has been reported with 6 weeks of RR [37].

As a result, in terms of advanced age ICU, as in all disease groups, COVID-19 patients also mean high usage of mechanical ventilation and high mortality. The limited number of studies presented above suggests that higher mortality rates are related to the number and nature of concomitant diseases rather than directly related to mechanical ventilation. Invasive mechanical ventilation is traditionally used for severe acute respiratory failure, including ARDS. As it is mentioned in the text, NIV, HFNO, and NIV/HFNO applications increase their value as an option. The available data are far from providing clear guidance on the choice of NIV or invasive MV in terms of the timing of the start of mechanical ventilation in elderly patients with COVID-19. At present, the decision to institute invasive mechanical ventilation (involving an endotracheal tube) is still based on physician judgment (clinical behavior influenced by oxygen saturation, dyspnea, respiratory rate, radiological imaging, etc.). With its basic starting point, the goal of not harming should cover both the timely and effective oxygenation and the least invasiveness of the work to be done. The available data suggest that it would be wise to decide on mechanical ventilation, first with clinical and then advanced laboratory evaluations. Likewise, it can be claimed that it would be appropriate to use invasive methods after starting support with noninvasive options at hand (NIV, HFNO). It should not be forgotten that at this stage, it may be necessary to make a choice considering the anatomical handicaps that may arise due to age or personal characteristics. To consider that invasive and noninvasive ventilation methods are complementary rather than alternatives, and invasive methods without hesitation should be adopted when the targeted physiological points cannot be reached.

References

1. https://www.who.int/emergencies/diseases/novel-coronavirus-2019.
2. https://www.worldometers.info/coronavirus/. https://blogs.bmj.com/bmj/2020/05/01/covid-19-a-complex-multisystem-clinical-syndrome/.
3. Clinical management of severe acute respiratory infection (SARI) when COVID-19 disease is suspected: Interim guidance. 13 March 2020. WHO reference number: WHO/2019-nCoV/clinical/2020.4.
4. Wang D, Hu B, Hu C, Zhu F, Liu X, Zhang J, Wang B, Xiang H, Cheng Z, Xiong Y, Zhao Y, Li Y, Wang X, Peng Z. Clinical characteristics of 138 hospitalized patients with 2019 novel coronavirus–infected pneumonia in Wuhan, China. JAMA. 2020;323:1061–9. https://doi.org/10.1001/jama.2020.1585.
5. Bhatraju PK, Ghassemieh BJ, Nichols M, Kim R, Jerome KR, Nalla AK, Greninger AL, Pipavath S, Wurfel MM, Evans L, Kritek PA, West TE, Luks A, Gerbino A, Dale CR, Goldman JD, O'Mahony S, Mikacenic C. Covid-19 in critically ill patients in the seattle region—case series. N Engl J Med. 2020;382:2012–22. https://doi.org/10.1056/NEJMoa2004500.
6. Zhou F, Yu T, Ronghui D, Fan G, Liu Y, Liu Z, Xiang J, Wang Y, Song B, Xiaoying G, Guan L, Wei Y, Li H, Wu X, Xu J, Shengjin T, Zhang Y, Chen H, Cao B. Clinical course and risk factors

for mortality of adult inpatients with COVID-19 in Wuhan, China: a retrospective cohort study. Lancet. 2020;395:P1054–62. https://doi.org/10.1016/S0140-6736(20)30566-3.

7. Grasselli G, Zangrillo A, Zanella A, Antonelli M, Cabrini L, Castelli A, Cereda D, Coluccello A, Foti G, Fumagalli R, Iotti G, Latronico N, Lorini L, Merler S, Natalini G, Piatti A, Ranieri MV, Scandroglio AM, Storti E, Cecconi M, Pesenti A, for the COVID-19 Lombardy ICU Network. Baseline characteristics and outcomes of 1591 patients infected with SARS-CoV-2 admitted to ICUs of the Lombardy Region, Italy. JAMA. 2020;323:1574–81. https://doi.org/10.1001/jama.2020.5394.

8. Xu Z, Shi L, Wang Y, Zhang J, Huang L, Zhang C, Liu S, Zhao P, Liu H, Zhu L, Tai Y, Bai C, Gao T, Song J, Xia P, Dong J, Zhao J, Wang F-S. Pathological findings of COVID-19 associated with acute respiratory distress syndrome. Lancet Respir Med. 2020;8:420–2. https://doi.org/10.1016/S2213-2600(20)30076-X.

9. Hanley B, Lucas SB, Youd E, Swift B, Osborn M. Autopsy in suspected COVID-19 cases. J Clin Pathol. 2020;73:1–4. https://doi.org/10.1136/jclinpath-2020-206522.

10. Barton LM, Duval EJ, Stroberg E, Ghosh S, Mukhopadhyay S. COVID-19 Autopsies, Oklahoma, USA. Am J Clin Pathol. 2020;153(6):725–33. https://doi.org/10.1093/AJCP/AQAA062.

11. Fox SE, Akmatbekov A, Harbert JL, Li G, Brown JQ, Vander Heide RS. Pulmonary and cardiac pathology in Covid-19: the first autopsy series from New Orleans. 2020; https://doi.org/10.1101/2020.04.06.20050575.

12. Ottestad W, Søvik S. COVID-19 patients with respiratory failure: what can we learn from aviation medicine? Br J Anaesth. 2020; https://doi.org/10.1016/j.bja.2020.04.012.

13. Tobin MJ. Basing respiratory management of coronavirus on physiological principles. Am J Respir Crit Care Med. 2020;201(11):1319–20. https://doi.org/10.1164/rccm.202004-1076ED.

14. Gattinoni L, Coppola S, Cressoni M, Busana M, Chiumello D. Covid-19 does not lead to a "typical" acute respiratory distress syndrome. Am J Respir Crit Care Med. 2020;201(10):1299–300. https://doi.org/10.1164/rccm.202003-0817LE.

15. Gattinoni L, Chiumello D, Caironi P, Busana M, Romitti F, Brazzi L, Camporota L. COVID-19 pneumonia: different respiratory treatment for different phenotypes? Intens Care Med. 2020;46:1099–102. https://doi.org/10.1007/s00134-020-06033-2.

16. Richardson S, Hirsch JS, Narasimhan M, Crawford JM, McGinn T, Davidson KW, and the Northwell COVID-19 Research Consortium. Presenting characteristics, comorbidities, and outcomes among 5700 patients hospitalized with COVID-19 in the New York City Area. JAMA. 2020;323(20):2052–9. https://doi.org/10.1001/jama.2020.6775.

17. Chen N, Zhou M, Dong X, Jieming Q, Gong F, Yang H, Yang Q, Wang J, Liu Y, Wei Y, Xia J'a, Yu T, Zhang X, Zhang L. Epidemiological and clinical characteristics of 99 cases of 2019 novel coronavirus pneumonia in Wuhan, China: a descriptive study. Lancet. 2020;395:P507–13.

18. Kang BJ, Koh YS, Lim CM, Huh JW, Baek SH, Han MJ, et al. Failure of high-flow nasal cannula therapy may delay intubation and increase mortality. Intensive Care Med. 2015;41:623–32.

19. Vosylius S, Sipylaite J, Ivaskevicius J. Determinants of outcome in elderly patients admitted to the intensive care unit. Age Ageing. 2005;34:157–62. https://doi.org/10.1093/ageing/afi037.

20. Esteban A, Anzueto A, Frutos-Vivar F, et al. Outcome of older patients receiving mechanical ventilation. Intensive Care Med. 2004;30:639–46.

21. Van den Noortgate N, Vogelaers D, Afschrift M, Colardyn F. Intensive care for very elderly patients: outcome and risk factors for in-hospital mortality. Age Ageing. 1999;28:253–6.

22. Farfel JM, Franca SA, Sitta MDC, Filho WJ, Carvalho CRR. Age, invasive ventilatory support and outcomes in elderly patients admitted to intensive care units. Age Ageing. 2009;38:515–20. https://doi.org/10.1093/ageing/afp119.

23. Xiao K, Liu B, Guan W, Yan P, Song L, Wang Y, Xie L. Prognostic analysis of elderly patients with multiple organ dysfunction syndrome undergoing invasive mechanical ventilation. J Healthc Eng. 2020;2020:6432048. https://doi.org/10.1155/2020/6432048.

24. Lieberman D, Nachshon L, Miloslavsky O, Dvorkin V, Shimoni A, Lieberman D. How do older ventilated patients fare? A survival/functional analysis of 641 ventilations. J Crit Care. 2009;24(3):340–6. https://doi.org/10.1016/j.jcrc.2009.01.015.

25. Scala R, Ciarleglio G, Maccari U, Granese V, Salerno L, Madioni C. Ventilator support and oxygen therapy in palliative and end-of-life Care in the Elderly. Turk Thorac J. 2020;21(1):54–60. https://doi.org/10.5152/TurkThoracJ.2020.201401.
26. Scala R, Pisani L. Noninvasive ventilation in acute respiratory failure: which recipe for success? Eur Respir Rev. 2018;27:pii: 180029.
27. Huang C-C, Muo C-H, Wu T-F, Chi T-Y, Shen T-C, Hsia T-C, Shih C-M. The application of non-invasive and invasive mechanical ventilation in the first episode of acute respiratory failure. Intern Emerg Med. 2020;30:1–9. https://doi.org/10.1007/s11739-020-02315-1.
28. Anon JM, Gómez-Tello V, González-Higueras E, Córcoles V, Quintana M, García de Lorenzo A, Onoro JJ, Martín-Delgado C, García-Fernández A, Marina L, Gordo F, Choperena G, Díaz-Alersi R, Montejo JC, López-Martínez J. Prognosis of elderly patients subjected to mechanical ventilation in the ICU. Med Int. 2013;37(3):149–55. https://doi.org/10.1016/j.medin.2012.03.014.
29. Lieberman D, Nachshon L, Miloslavsky O, Dvorkin V, Shimoni A, Zelinger J, Friger M, Lieberman D. Elderly patients undergoing mechanical ventilation in and out of intensive care units: a comparative, prospective study of 579 ventilations. Crit Care. 2010;14:R48.
30. Barnato AE, Albert SM, Angus DC, Lave JR, Degenholtz HB. Disability among elderly survivors of mechanical ventilation. Am J Respir Crit Care Med. 2011;183:1037–42. https://doi.org/10.1164/rccm.201002-0301OC.
31. Cruz RS, Villarejo F, Figueroa A, Corte's-Jofre M, Gagliardi J, Navarrete M. Mortality in critically ill elderly individuals receiving mechanical ventilation. Respir Care. 2019;64(4):473–83. https://doi.org/10.4187/respcare.06586.
32. Li Q, Zhang J, Wan X. Analysis of characteristics and related risk factors of prognosis in elderly and young adult patients with acute respiratory distress syndrome. Zhonghua Wei Zhong Bing Ji Jiu Yi Xue. 2014;26(11):794–8.
33. Duke GJ, Barker A, Knott CI, Santamaria JD. Outcomes of older people receiving intensive care in Victoria. Med J Aust. 2014;200(6):323–6.
34. Suchyta MR, Clemmer TP, Elliott CG, Orme JF Jr, Weaver LK. The adult respiratory distress syndrome. A report of survival and modifying factors. Chest. 1992;101(4):1074–9.
35. Zilberberg MD, Epstein SK. Acute lung injury in the medical ICU: comorbid conditions, age, etiology, and hospital outcome. Am J Respir Crit Care Med. 1998;157(4 Pt 1):1159–64.
36. Liu K, Chen Y, Lin R, Han K. Clinical features of COVID-19 in elderly patients: a comparison with young and middle-aged patients. J Inf Secur. 2020;80:e14–8. https://doi.org/10.1016/j.jinf.2020.03.005.
37. Liu K, Zhang W, Yang Y, Zhang J, Li Y, Chen Y. Respiratory rehabilitation in elderly patients with COVID-19: a randomized controlled study. Complement Ther Clin Pract. 2020;39:101166.

The Role of ECMO

16

Mohammed D. Alahmari

16.1 Background

Extracorporeal membrane oxygenation (ECMO) is a form of cardiopulmonary support for patients with severe acute hypoxemic respiratory failure (AHRF). ECMO involves the use of a circuit to divert cardiac output through an artificial gas-exchange device in order to facilitate the removal of carbon dioxide and the addition of oxygen [1]. There are two types of ECMO, which differ depending on which vessels are cannulated for the circuit: veno-arterial (V-A) ECMO and veno-venous (V-V) ECMO. The promising results [2] and experience acquired during the 2009 H1N1 influenza pandemic [3] led many centers to adopt ECMO as a rescue therapy for acute respiratory distress syndrome (ARDS) patients who do not respond to conventional mechanical ventilation [2]. Regardless of the continuing debate and conflicting data surrounding its use, ECMO remains a reasonable alternative supportive therapy to conventional mechanical ventilation strategies [4].

ECMO is a specialized intensive technique that requires the use of extremely limited resources. It is generally recommended to only use this technique as a rescue therapy for carefully selected patients [5]. Controversial evidence has been reported concerning clinical outcomes of severe respiratory distress syndrome and refractory hypoxemia [3, 6, 7].

M. D. Alahmari (✉)
Department of Respiratory Care, Prince Sultan Military College of Health Sciences, Dammam, Saudi Arabia

Eastern Province Health Cluster, Dammam, Saudi Arabia
e-mail: Mohamed.alahmari@kfsh.med.sa

© The Editor(s) (if applicable) and The Author(s), under exclusive license to   153
Springer Nature Switzerland AG 2020
N. Vargas, A. M. Esquinas (eds.), *Covid-19 Airway Management and Ventilation Strategy for Critically Ill Older Patients*, https://doi.org/10.1007/978-3-030-55621-1_16

16.2   Indications of ECMO

For the most critically ill patients, ECMO only provides support to the lungs and the heart but not to other organs. In the COVID-19 pandemic, ECMO should not be used as a first-line resource or be rushed into service in such a manner that would overwhelm clinicians and healthcare systems. Currently, ECMO is indicated for critically ill ARDS patients with severe refractory hypoxemia (PaO_2/FIO_2 < 80 mmHg on ≥90% FiO_2), severe retention of CO_2 ($PaCO_2$ > 80 mmHg), severe barotrauma with air leakage, and/or inability to achieve a plateau pressure ≤ 30 cmH_2O [8].

The WHO has recommended the use of ECMO for suspected eligible COVID-19 patients with ARDS in well-specialized healthcare centers [9]. ECMO utilization data from previous outbreaks of influenza A (H1N1) in 2009 are not clear. In New Zealand and Australia, the estimated rate of ECMO use was 2.6 cases per million, whereas in Saudi Arabia, ECMO was used in 5.8% of critically ill patients with MERS-CoV-related ARDS [2, 10].

ECMO should be avoided in patients who are advanced in age, have comorbidities, and are experiencing multiple organ failure. Table 16.1 lists the relative and absolute contraindications for ECMO in COVID-19 patients [11].

Table 16.1 Contraindications of using ECMO with COVID-19 adult patients

Relative contraindications	Absolute contraindications

• Age ≥ 65 years
• Obesity body mass index ≥40
• Immunocompromised patients
• Lack of legal medical decision maker
• Advanced chronic underlying systolic heart failure
• High-dose vasopressor requirement (and not under consideration for V-A or V-VA ECMO)
	• Elderly age
	• Clinical frailty scale category ≥3
	• Under mechanical ventilation >10 days
	Significant underlying comorbidities:
	  Chronic kidney disease ≥ III
	  Cirrhosis
	  Dementia
	  Baseline neurologic disease which would preclude rehabilitation potential
	  Disseminated malignancy
	  Advanced lung disease
	  Uncontrolled diabetes with chronic end-organ dysfunction
	  Severe deconditioning
	  Protein-energy malnutrition
	  Severe peripheral vascular disease
	  Other pre-existing life-limiting medical condition
	  Non-ambulatory or unable to perform activities
	• Severe multiple organ failure
	• Severe acute neurologic injury
	• Uncontrolled bleeding
	• Anticoagulation
	• Inability to accept blood products
	• Ongoing cardiopulmonary resuscitation

16.3   ECMO Management

The role of ECMO in the management of the COVID-19 pandemic remains unclear despite the increased use of ECMO [12, 13]. ECMO can be helpful as a supportive therapy but has not yet yielded any definitive outcomes in the management of acute hypoxemic respiratory failure in selected COVID-19 patients [14]. During this pandemic, it is especially important to consider elderly patients and patients with comorbidities as mortality rates increase. Selection criteria are important to identify those who will benefit most from ECMO; for example, relocation of resources, young age, and single organ failure are crucially important to successful outcomes of ECMO use [11].

In mechanically ventilated patients with COVID-19, ECMO should only be considered in a selected population of severe ARDS patients [5]. However, no clinical trials have been conducted to examine the outcomes of ECMO use with COVID-19 patients. A retrospective observational study in Wuhan, China, revealed that out of 52 critically ill adult patients, six (11.5%) received prone positioning and EMCO; however, the clinical outcomes of this study have not yet been reported [15]. During the Middle East respiratory syndrome-related coronavirus (MERS-CoV) epidemic in 2012, a retrospective cohort study by a Saudi group reported lower in-hospital mortality (65 vs. 100%, $P = 0.02$) in 17 patients receiving ECMO versus 17 patients receiving conventional therapy [16]. Another study showed that the PaO_2/FIO_2 ratios of patients receiving ECMO improved 7 and 14 days after ICU admission, necessitating less use of norepinephrine; this result suggested that ECMO is a recommend selective rescue therapy for MERS-CoV patients with refractory hypoxemia [16].

V-V ECMO is recommended for COVID-19 patients when all standardized therapies for ARDS, particularly prone positioning, have been maximally utilized [1]. It is clear that ARDS in COVID-19 is not yet well understood, and mechanical ventilation strategies applied prior to initiation of V-V ECMO may affect clinical outcomes [17]. Therefore, specific mechanical ventilation management strategies have not yet been presented for COVID-19. However, V-A ECMO is recommended for patients before multiple organ failure occurs [11] and in selected cases of refractory cardiogenic shock [18]. There is no clear consensus on the proper mechanical ventilation strategy for ECMO with ARDS patients. Two randomized trials of ECMO for ARDS patients could serve as useful sources of mechanical ventilation strategies (EOLIA [19]; plateau pressure $\leq$ 24 cmH$_2$O; positive end-expiratory pressure (PEEP) $\leq$ 10 cmH$_2$O; respiratory rate = 10–30 breaths per min) and ECMO strategies for severe adult respiratory failure (CESAR [6]; peak inspiratory pressure = 20–25 cmH$_2$O; PEEP $\leq$10 cmH$_2$O; respiratory rate = 10 breaths per min).

In one of the largest case series, most critically ill COVID-19 patients appeared to have developed cardiac shock or arrhythmias; however, a lack of knowledge concerning multiorgan failure may have limited ECMO utilization [20]. Given the limited amount of data concerning this virus and its mechanism of causing death, ECMO use has been limited to selected patients with unknown outcomes. The enormous, increasing number of infectious patients produced by this outbreak is expected to charge intensive care units with significant challenges and resource consumption. In order to arrive at a decision of whether to use ECMO during this pandemic, it is essential to balance the risk-to-benefit ratio. ECMO is not likely to benefit COVID-19 patients with septic shock and refractory multiorgan failure [21] because of the severity of illness exhibited by such patients. However, other limitations presented by this pandemic have included shortages of trained staff, equipment, disposables, and proper isolation room infrastructure. The decision of whether to initiate ECMO for the treatment of COVID-19 [22] should be made on a local, case-by-case basis and should depend on hospital resources. During this pandemic, healthcare providers and younger patients should be prioritized in the selection of ECMO candidates in cases of COVID-19 infection.

16.4 ECMO Preparedness

ECMO preparedness is important during outbreaks such as the COVID-19 pandemic. Remanathan et al. [23] categorized organizational ECMO preparedness services into four types: personnel, equipment, facilities, and systems. Important elements of planning for ECMO service utilization in the COVID-19 pandemic include maintenance of multidisciplinary ECMO teams specialized and trained for this service; tracking of equipment and supply records; identification of resources; minimization of waste; clustering of infected patients with strict precautions and procedures/protocols for waste disposal and patient transport; and proper systems for communications, coordination, reporting, resource allocation, and quality assurance. Protocols for ECMO weaning should be standardized in healthcare centers [24] and accompanied by proper decannulation and rehabilitation with strict infection control measures.

16.5 Ethical Issues

Ethical considerations present challenges for the use of ECMO in a pandemic [25, 26]. During the current outbreak of COVID-19, the potential benefits and outcomes of implementing ECMO are difficult to measure due to the evolving, infectious nature of the disease. Given the current shortages of machines, trained staff, and resources, the selection of patients for ECMO presents ethical dilemmas in the absence of strong evidence for the benefits of ECMO use. Dedicated hospital ethics committees for pandemics should be prepared to interfere in such challenging scenarios as those presented by the surge of COVID-19 [27, 28].

16.6 Conclusions and Recommendations

Global collaboration is needed to contain COVID-19 and understand the effects of COVID-19 infection on the lungs and development of ARDS phenotypes. Such understanding is necessary to measure the benefits and outcomes of ECMO use during outbreaks of infectious diseases. The following are summarizing the recommendations of using ECMO with COVID-19 pandemic:

- There is a lack or paucity of high quality of evidence for ECMO use in COVID-19 pandemic.
- ECMO is a recommended rescue therapy in COVID-19 pandemic in established centers, with responsible utilization in case of crisis capacity [29].
- Creation of ECMO networking at national and regional is essential during outbreaks to maximize and share benefits through proper coordination such as staff in case of understaffing in other local centers, equipment, and communication for clinical experiences.
- ECMO should be the last therapy to initiate with ARDS after maximizing all other therapies including prone positioning.
- Rational decisions are crucially needed to avoid or timing for some procedures while COVID-19 patient on ECMO to protect staff from unnecessary exposure.
- Ethical dilemmas are significant during a pandemic. Involvement of supportive and palliative care teams are important in particular prior to cannulation [11]. Staff also need debriefing to deal in such pandemics and crisis with the support of or access of psychology and psychiatric team.

References

1. Brodie D, Slutsky A, Combes A. Extracorporeal life support for adults with respiratory failure and related indications. JAMA. 2019;322(6):557–68.
2. Australia and New Zealand Extracorporeal Membrane Oxygenation (ANZ ECMO) Influenza Investigators, Davies A, Jones D, et al. Extracorporeal Membrane Oxygenation for 2009 Influenza A(H1N1) acute respiratory distress syndrome. JAMA. 2009;302(17):1888–95.
3. Pham T, Combes A, Rozé H, Chevret S, Mercat A, Roch A, et al. Extracorporeal membrane oxygenation for pandemic influenza A (H1N1)–induced acute respiratory distress syndrome. Am J Respir Crit Care Med. 2013;187(3):276–85.
4. Park P, Dalton H, Bartlett R. Point: efficacy of extracorporeal membrane oxygenation in 2009 influenza A (H1N1). Chest. 2010;138(4):776–8.
5. Alhazzani W, Moller M, Arabi Y, Loeb M, Gong M, Fan E, et al. Surviving Sepsis campaign: guidelines on the management of critically ill adults with coronavirus disease 2019 (COVID-19). Intensive Care Med. 2020;48:e440.
6. Peek G, Mugford M, Tiruvoipati R, Wilson A, Allen E, Thalanany M, et al. Efficacy and economic assessment of conventional ventilatory support versus extracorporeal membrane oxygenation for severe adult respiratory failure (CESAR): a multicentre randomised controlled trial. Lancet. 2009;374(9698):1351–63.
7. Munshi L, Walkey A, Goligher E, Pham T, Uleryk E, Fan E. Venovenous extracorporeal membrane oxygenation for acute respiratory distress syndrome: a systematic review and meta-analysis. Lancet Respir Med. 2019;7(2):163–72.
8. Combes A, Bréchot N, Luyt C, Schmidt M. Extracorporeal membrane oxygenation. Curr Opin Crit Care. 2017;23(1):60–5.
9. https://www.who.int/docs/default-source/coronaviruse/clinical-management-of-novel-cov.pdf. Accessed 29 Apr 2020.

10. Arabi Y, Al-Omari A, Mandourah Y, Al-Hameed F, Sindi A, Alraddadi B, et al. Critically ill patients with the Middle East respiratory syndrome. Crit Care Med. 2017;45(10):1683–95.

11. www.elso.org/Resources/Guidelines.aspx. Accessed 26 Apr 2020.

12. www.elso.org/Registry/FullCOVID19RegistryDashboard.aspx. Accessed 24 Apr 2020.

13. www.euroelso.net/covid-19/covid-19-survey/. Accessed 27 Apr 2020.

14. Goligher E, Tomlinson G, Hajage D, Wijeysundera D, Fan E, Jüni P, et al. Extracorporeal Membrane Oxygenation for severe acute respiratory distress syndrome and posterior probability of mortality benefit in a post hoc Bayesian analysis of a randomized clinical trial. JAMA. 2018;320(21):2251–9.

15. Yang X, Yu Y, Xu J, Shu H, Xia J, Liu H, et al. Clinical course and outcomes of critically ill patients with SARS-CoV-2 pneumonia in Wuhan, China: a single-centered, retrospective, observational study. Lancet Respir Med. 2020;8:P475–81.

16. Alshahrani M, Sindi A, Alshamsi F, Al-Omari A, El Tahan M, Alahmadi B, et al. Extracorporeal membrane oxygenation for severe Middle East respiratory syndrome coronavirus. Ann Intensive Care. 2018;8(1):3.

17. Schmidt M, Pham T, Arcadipane A, Agerstrand C, Ohshimo S, Pellegrino V, et al. Mechanical ventilation management during Extracorporeal Membrane Oxygenation for acute respiratory distress syndrome. An international multicenter prospective cohort. Am J Respir Crit Care Med. 2019;200(8):1002–12.

18. Reyentovich A, Barghash M, Hochman J. Management of refractory cardiogenic shock. Nat Rev Cardiol. 2016;13(8):481–92.

19. Mi M, Matthay M, Morris A. Extracorporeal Membrane Oxygenation for severe acute respiratory distress syndrome. N Engl J Med. 2018;379(9):884–7.

20. Wang D, Hu B, Hu C, Zhu F, Liu X, Zhang J, et al. Clinical characteristics of 138 hospitalized patients with 2019 novel coronavirus–infected pneumonia in Wuhan, China. JAMA. 2020;323(11):1061–9.

21. MacLaren G, Fisher D, Brodie D. Preparing for the Most critically ill patients with COVID-19. JAMA. 2020;323(13):E1–2.

22. Bartlett R, Ogino M, Brodie D, McMullan D, Lorusso R, MacLaren G, et al. Initial ELSO Guidance Document. ASAIO J. 2020;66(5):472–4.

23. Ramanathan K, Antognini D, Combes A, Paden M, Zakhary B, Ogino M, et al. Planning and provision of ECMO services for severe ARDS during the COVID-19 pandemic and other outbreaks of emerging infectious diseases. Lancet Respir Med. 2020;8:518.

24. Vasques F, Romitti F, Gattinoni L, Camporota L. How I wean patients from veno-venous extracorporeal membrane oxygenation. Crit Care. 2019;23(1):316.

25. Abrams D, Pham T, Burns K, Combes A, Curtis J, Mueller T, et al. Practice patterns and ethical considerations in the management of venovenous extracorporeal membrane oxygenation patients. Crit Care Med. 2019;47(10):1346–55.

26. Abrams D, Curtis J, Prager K, Garan A, Hastie J, Brodie D. Ethical considerations for mechanical support. Anesthesiol Clin. 2019;37(4):661–73.

27. Ramanathan K, Cove M, Caleb M, Teoh K, Maclaren G. Ethical dilemmas of adult ECMO: emerging conceptual challenges. J Cardiothorac Vasc Anesth. 2015;29(1):229–33.

28. Bein T, Brodie D. Understanding ethical decisions for patients on extracorporeal life support. Intensive Care Med. 2017;43(10):1510–1.

29. Hick J, Barbera J, Kelen G. Refining surge capacity: conventional, contingency, and crisis capacity. Disaster Med Public Health Prep. 2009;3(S1):S59–67.

The Role of HFNC

17

Giuseppe Fiorentino, Maurizia Lanza, Anna Annunziata, and Pasquale Imitazione

Abbreviations

ARF	Acute respiratory failure
COVID-19	Coronavirus disease 2019
HFNC	High-flow nasal cannula
O_2 therapy	Oxygen therapy
PP	Prone position

17.1 Introduction

Coronavirus disease 2019 (COVID-19) is a respiratory tract infection caused by a newly emergent coronavirus, which was first recognized in Wuhan, China, in December 2019. Modes of transmission of disease are direct inhalation of infected droplets (produced during coughing or sneezing by infected person) and direct contact with surfaces and fomites soiled by infected respiratory secretions. Special condition (cardiopulmonary resuscitation, endotracheal intubation, open suctioning, bronchoscopy, nebulization and use of noninvasive ventilation) can lead to aerosol generation and propagation [1].

Currently, the World Health Organization (WHO) has defined the infection as a global pandemic. Acute respiratory infection due to 2019 novel coronavirus (2019-nCoV) is now known as novel coronavirus-infected pneumonia (NCIP) [2]. While most people with COVID-19 develop only mild or uncomplicated illness, approximately 14% develop severe disease that requires hospitalization and oxygen

G. Fiorentino (✉) · M. Lanza · A. Annunziata · P. Imitazione
Unit of Respiratory Physiopathology, Monaldi Hospital, Naples, Italy

© The Editor(s) (if applicable) and The Author(s), under exclusive license to Springer Nature Switzerland AG 2020
N. Vargas, A. M. Esquinas (eds.), *Covid-19 Airway Management and Ventilation Strategy for Critically Ill Older Patients*, https://doi.org/10.1007/978-3-030-55621-1_17

support, and 5% require admission to an intensive care unit (ICU). The conventional oxygen therapy via nasal cannula or face mask is important for the management of respiratory failure during the initial phase, while the request is noninvasive ventilation (NIV) or invasive mechanical ventilation for the most serious cases. However, these procedures may generate respiratory droplets.

17.2   Rationale Use of HFNC

High-flow nasal cannula (HFNC) is increasingly used in the management of chronic and acute respiratory failure (ARF) caused by various different clinical conditions. High-flow nasal cannula (HFNC) oxygen therapy is a technique that can deliver a FiO_2 up to 1.0 by supplying warm, humidified oxygen through a nasal cannula. The system includes a blender, active humidifier, single heated tube, and nasal cannula. Recently, various attempts have been made to apply HFNC oxygen therapy to patients with ARF. Although the technique does not reduce the need for endotracheal intubation or mortality compared to conventional oxygen therapy or noninvasive ventilation (NIV), it has advantages such as patient comfort and tolerability [3]. The greater flow corresponds to the patient's demand, reduces anatomical dead space by decreasing the extent of breathing and provides positive pressure in the upper airways [4]. In patients with acute hypoxemic respiratory failure, HFNC reduced inspiratory effort and improved oxygenation and dynamic compliance [5]. HFNC carbon dioxide tension reduction and the effect is dependent on flow and leaks through airway flushing and functional dead space reduction.

17.3   Usefulness to HFNC Use in COVID Patients

The high-flow nasal cannula (HFNC) is commonly used in patients with hypoxemic respiratory failure [6]. Due to a limited number of ventilators available in hospitals, the use of HFNC may be a good option to use before patients develop severe hypoxemic respiratory failure. The new coronavirus disease (COVID-19) caused severe acute respiratory syndrome that may involve the use of countless resources. The patients who develop moderate-to-severe respiratory failure who require oxygen supplementation devices such as lung ventilators and high-flow nasal cannula (HFNC). The World Health Organization (WHO) has published a guide on managing severe respiratory infections when COVID-19 is suspected [7]. Using evidence from several recently published studies [8], the WHO guide claims that HFNC does not create a widespread dispersion of exhaled air and therefore should be associated with a low risk of transmission of respiratory viruses. This document also recommended to wear a standard medical mask if the healthcare provider is located within 2 m from the patient and there is a physical separation of the bed at least 1 m. However, the secondary inhalation of emissions released by patients with COVID-19 using HFNC is a real concern. It leads to the risk of aerosol virus dispersion since HFNC does not have a closed circuit, a difference of the pulmonary ventilator.

Previous studies presented show a low risk of airborne transmission HFNC when you get a good adaptation of the interface [9]. The HFNC safe use in patients with coronavirus and the risk/benefit ratio for the delivery of aerosols through HFNC has not been studied. Previous research has reported that an increase in the flow has reduced fugitive emissions and the size of the aerosol particles during therapy [10]. Doctors need to place surgical masks on the faces of infected patients during the HFNC and administer therapy with aerosols in a local negative pressure. Respiratory therapists should also wear personal protective equipment, including an N95 respirator, goggles/visor, double gloves, dress or apron if the gown is not fluid resistant [11].

17.4 Bio-aerosol Dispersion during HFNC

The primary strategy for COVID-19 patients is supportive care, including oxygen therapy for hypoxemic patients, in which high-flow nasal cannula (HFNC) was reported as effective in improving oxygenation. Among patients with acute hypoxemic respiratory failure, HFNC was proven to avoid intubation compared to conventional oxygen device [12]. But, there is an important preoccupation that HFNC may increase bio-aerosol dispersion in the surroundings due to the high gas flow used. The increased dispersion might favor transmission of infectious agents (such as COVID-19) carried in aerosol droplets generated by the infected patient [13]. In the western world there is a tendency to avoid HFNC in COVID-19 patients. This translates into an increased recourse to early intubation and consequently to a higher incidence of potential damages associated with sedation, infections also due to prolonged stay of intensive care units. Furthermore, let us not forget that the intubation procedure itself is a high-risk situation for viral exposure. Early intubation increases the demand for fans, contributing to the critical shortage reported worldwide. Avoiding or delaying the invasive mechanical ventilation could substantially reduce the immediate demand of fans. Therefore, we aimed to discuss the scientific evidence supporting the dispersal risk of bio-aerosols induced by HFNC in COVID-19 context. Hui et al. in a comparison study of exhaled air dispersion during high-flow nasal cannula therapy versus CPAP via different masks claim that the dispersion distance of the exhaled air during the application of HFNC at 60 L min^{-1} is less than that from the application of the CPAP through the commonly used nasal pillows. However, losses to 620 mm laterally may occur in the presence of a loose connection between HFNC and the interface tube [8]. As aerosol generated by patient's cough contains particles from 0.1 to 100 μm, clinical studies are demanded to truly evaluate aerosol dispersion, particularly the aerosol dynamics during physiological exhalation and cough. In vitro and clinical studies have demonstrated that the application of a simple surgical mask on patients significantly reduces the creep age distance and the bio-aerosol infected with virus at 20 cm distance from patients while coughing [14]. Surgical mask can be worn by the patient only when they are oxygenated through a nasal cannula (standard nasal cannula or HFNC) but not when using simple oxygen masks, non-respirable or Venturi [15]. Taken together, compared to oxygen with a mask, the use of HFNC neither increases nor the dispersion nor the microbiological contamination in the environment; the possibility for the patient to wear a surgical mask over HFNC to reduce the transmission of aerosol during coughing or sneezing represents a further advantage. However, given the high HFNC effectiveness to oxygenate the patient, carefully monitoring the use of HFNC is essential for COVID-19 patients in order to avoid delayed intubation, respiratory rate, pulse oximetry, and clinical examination. A considerable number of clinicians during the COVID-19 pandemic have been infected. This figure has increased concerns about requiring the generation of aerosol, and therefore the current tendency is to avoid HFNC. But the generation of scientific evidence and dispersal of bio-aerosols through HFNC show a risk similar to standard oxygen masks. The use of HFNC with a surgical mask on the patient's face may then be a reasonable practice that can be beneficial to patients hypoxemic COVID-19 and avoid intubation [16].

17.5   Self-Proning with High-Flow Nasal Cannula

More serious cases of COVID-19 lead to acute respiratory distress syndrome (ARDS) and this is one of the hallmark features of critical COVID-19 cases. ARDS can be directly life threatening because it is associated with low blood oxygenation levels and can result in organ failure [17]. There are no generally recognized effective treatments for COVID-19, but treatments are urgently needed. In the ARDS treatments more studies suggest the prone position (PP) during the ventilation of COVID-19 patient. The PP increases the media ratio of arterial oxygen tension to the fraction of inspired oxygen (PaO_2/FiO_2) by +35 mmHg and decreases mortality in moderate-to-severe ARDS. Actually, PP was only recommended in severe ARDS with $PaO_2/FiO_2 < 100$ mmHg, and his use is less than 33% of severe ARDS patients [18]. Both NIV and HFNC techniques work with two different mechanisms, and from a theoretical and physiological point of view, they open collapsed alveoli and increase residual functional capacity. In this way, improving ventilation-perfusion matching and reducing intrapulmonary shunt, as well as improving lung compliance, thus decreasing the respiratory load [19]. In this regard, combining PP with these noninvasive respiratory supports in ARDS may result in better physiological effects on ventilation–perfusion mismatch and greater homogeneity in ARDS mechanics while receiving positive pressure support. Based on these mechanisms, Ding et al. studied, in a prospective observational study, the idea that early use of PP combined with either NIV or HFNC avoided the need for intubation in patients with severe ARDS. They also rated how PP combined with HFNC or NIV provided the PaO_2/FiO_2 compared to only HFNC or NIV support, and the safety of PP therapy in wakefulness, in ARDS patients [20]. This study revealed that early PP combined with HFNC/NIV may avoid the need for intubation in up to half of the patients with moderate-to-severe ARDS; when PP was added, PaO_2/FiO_2 increased by 25–35 mmHg compared with the prior HFNC or NIV; and PP was safely performed and well tolerated by the moderate ARDS patients. Prone positioning may decrease the need for intubation and even mortality by improving the oxygenation of ARDS [18]. When PP was performed in intubated ARDS patients, high dose of sedation or even neuromuscular blockers may be needed. The addition of PP showed an increase for oxygenation in most cases. The hospital policies that address early intubation of COVID-19 patients will accelerate the employment of resources in an intensive care unit (ICU), including fans, sedative drugs, and human resources. Emerging evidence recommend that COVID-19 patients develop atypical acute respiratory distress syndrome (ARDS) with relatively preserved lung mechanics despite severe hypoxemia due to shunt fraction [21]. It is additionally known that prone positioning can improve oxygenation and reduce shunt fraction [22]. Current recommendation is therefore to suggest to patients who do not exhibit an increased work of breathing use of HFNC to meet the oxygen demands and instruct them to manage their position regardless of the body. Total time of pronation should be about 16–18 h/day (including 8–10 h while sleeping at night). Gattinoni et al. described two time-related phenotypes of COVID-19 pneumonia. Initially, many patients experience severe hypoxemia in the absence of dyspnea and maintenance of lung compliance with low ventilation/perfusion (V/Q) ratio (defined as L-phenotype). Over time, the lung picture ends in a classic form of ARDS with low lung compliance (defined as phenotype H) [23]. They proposed that the reason for hypoxemia in phenotype L is the dysregulation of lung perfusion and loss of hypoxic vasoconstriction. The prone position is more uniform distribution of lung tissue between dorsal and ventral floors that represent a more uniform honeycomb architecture. In addition, it also brings a more uniform distribution of pulmonary perfusion [24]. Therefore, in the early stages the combined use of HFNC with PP restores hypoxic pulmonary vasoconstriction, which is compromised at low oxygen levels and prevents worsening of dyspnea while a redistribution of lung tissue with auto proning alters the pulmonary stress-strain relationships and intrathoracic forces, slowing down the formation of pulmonary edema and progression of disease from phenotype L to H. This care approach would have importance in limited-resource applications in countries where there may not be sophisticated intensive care techniques available.

17.6 Conclusion

Due to a limited number of ventilators available in hospitals, the use of HFNC may be a good option to use before patients develop severe hypoxemic respiratory failure. The new coronavirus disease (COVID-19) caused by severe acute respiratory syndrome coronavirus-2 involves the use of countless resources. Taken together, compared to oxygen with a mask, the use of HFNC neither increases nor the dispersion nor the microbiological contamination in the environment; the possibility for the patient to wear a surgical mask over HFNC to reduce the transmission of aerosol during coughing or sneezing represents a further advantage. In the early stages the combined use of HFNC with PP represents a further weapon at our disposal to manage the COVID patient especially in limited-resource countries and for older patients.

References

1. Interim U.S. Center for Disease Control and Prevention. Guidance for Risk Assessment and Public Health Management of Healthcare Personnel with Potential Exposure in a Healthcare Setting to Patients with Coronavirus Disease (COVID-19); 2020. https://www.cdc.gov/coronavirus/2019-ncov/hcp/guidance-risk-assesment-hcp.html.
2. Zhou P, Yang XL, Wang XG, et al. A pneumonia outbreak associated with a new coronavirus of probable bat origin. Nature. 2020 Mar;579(7798):270–3.
3. Monro-Somerville T, Sim M, Ruddy J, et al. The effect of high-flow nasal cannula oxygen therapy on mortality and intubation rate in acute respiratory failure: a systematic review and meta-analysis. Crit Care Med. 2017;45(4):e449–56.
4. Moller W, Feng S, Domanski U, et al. Nasal high flow reduces dead space. J Appl Physiol. 2017;122(1):191–7.
5. Mauri T, Alban L, Turrini C, et al. Optimum support by high-flow nasal cannula in acute hypoxemic respiratory failure: effects of increasing flow rates. Intensive Care Med. 2017;43(10):1453–63.
6. Frat JP, Coudroy R, Marjanovic N, et al. High-flow nasal oxygen therapy and noninvasive ventilation in the management of acute hypoxemic respiratory failure. Ann Transl Med. 2017;5(14):297.
7. World Health Organization. Clinical management of severe acute respiratory infection when novel coronavirus (2019-nCoV) infection is suspected. Interim guidance. Available from: https://www.who.int/publications-detail/clinical-management-of-severe-acute respiratory-infection-when-novel-coronavirus-(ncov) infection-is-suspected. Accessed Mar 2020.
8. Hui DS, Chow BK, Lo T, et al. Exhaled air dispersion during high-flow nasal cannula therapy versus CPAP via different masks. Eur Respir J. 2019;53(4):1802339.
9. Leung C, Joynt G, Gomersall C. Comparison of high-flow nasal cannula versus oxygen face mask for environmental bacterial contamination in critically ill pneumonia patients: a randomized controlled crossover trial. J Hosp Infect. 2019;101(1):84–7.
10. McGrath JA, O'Toole C, Bennett G, et al. Investigation of fugitive aerosols released into the environment during high-flow therapy. Pharmaceutics. 2019;11(6):254.
11. Association CM. Expert consensus on protective measures related to respiratory therapy in patients with severe and critical coronavirus infection. Chin J Tuberc Respir Dis. 2020;17:E020.
12. Rochwerg B, Granton D, Wang DX, et al. High flow nasal cannula compared with conventional oxygen therapy for acute hypoxemic respiratory failure: a systematic review and meta-analysis. Intensive Care Med. 2019;45(5):563–72.
13. Ong SWX, Tan YK, Chia PY, et al. Air, surface environmental, and personal protective equipment contamination by severe acute respiratory syndrome coronavirus 2 (SARS-CoV-2) from a symptomatic patient. JAMA. 2020;323:1610–2. https://doi.org/10.1001/jama.2020.3227.
14. Hui DS, Chow BK, Chu L, et al. Exhaled air dispersion during coughing with and without wearing a surgical or N95 mask. PLoS One. 2012;7(12):e50845.
15. Johnson DF, Druce JD, Birch C, et al. A quantitative assessment of the efficacy of surgical and N95 masks to filter influenza virus in patients with acute influenza infection. Clin Infect Dis. 2009;49(2):275–7.
16. Li J, Fink JB, Ehrmann S. High-flow nasal cannula for COVID-19 patients: low risk of bioaerosol dispersion. Eur Respir J. 2020; https://doi.org/10.1183/13993003.00892-2020.
17. Arabi YM, Fowler R, Hayden FG. Critical care management of adults with community acquired severe respiratory viral infection. Intensive Care Med. 2020;46(2):315–28.
18. Guerin C, Beuret P, Constantin JM, et al. A prospective international observationalprevalence study on prone positioning of ARDS patients: the APRONET (ARDSprone position network) study. Intensive Care Med. 2018;44(1):22–37.

19. Frat JP, Brugiere B, Ragot S, et al. Sequential application of oxygen therapy via high-flow nasal cannula and noninvasive ventilation in acute respiratory failure: an observational pilot study. Respir Care. 2015;60(2):170–8.
20. Lin D, Wang L, Ma W, et al. Efficacy and safety of early prone positioning combined with HFNC or NIV in moderate to severe ARDS: a multi-center prospective cohort study. Crit Care. 2020;24(1):28.
21. Gattinoni L, Coppola S, Cressoni M, et al. Covid-19 does not lead to a "typical" acute respiratory distress syndrome. Am J Respir Crit Care Med. 2020;201(10):1299–300.
22. Matthay MA, Aldrich JM, Gotts JE. Treatment for severe acute respiratory distress syndrome from COVID-19. Lancet Respir Med. 2020;8(5):433–4.
23. Gattinoni L, Chiumello D, Caironi P, et al. COVID-19 pneumonia: different respiratory treatment for different phenotypes? Intensive Care Med. 2020;46(6):1099–102.
24. Kallet RH. A comprehensive review of prone position in ARDS. Respir Care. 2015;60(11):1660–87.

The Problem of Aerosolization

18

Hadeer S. Harb, Yasmin M. Madney,
Mohamed E. Abdelrahim, and Haitham Saeed

18.1 Introduction

Transmission of COVID-19 is primarily through droplets (only short distances) and fomite spread (e.g., clothing, equipment, furniture) that can become contaminated by the virus [1]. In contrast, aerosols are composed of much smaller fluid particles that can remain suspended in the air for prolonged periods [2]. Current evidence suggests that coronaviruses can survive in the aerosol within fluid particles under certain conditions [3, 4]. Some events can potentially lead to aerosolization of virally contaminated body fluid (aerosol-generating procedures "AGPs"), including coughing/sneezing/expectorating, NIV, HFNC, jet ventilation, delivery of nebulized medications via simple face mask, cardiopulmonary resuscitation (before tracheal intubation) and tracheal extubation [5, 6]. A higher risk of viral aerosolization was reported with tracheal suction (without a closed system), tracheal intubation, laryngoscopy, bronchoscopy/gastroscopy and tracheostomy/cricothyroidotomy [6]. Thus, these procedures carry a potential increased risk of nosocomial infection to healthcare workers (HCWs) and COVID-19 has now been classified as a high consequence infectious disease (HCID), emphasizing the significant risk to HCWs and the healthcare system [1].

18.2 Protective Strategies (Table 18.1)

Many protective strategies should be applied during the management of COVID-19 patients to protect HCWs. Helmet interface covering the entire patient head is advisable to be used for NIV delivery, especially with long-term therapy [7]. Unfortunately,

H. S. Harb · Y. M. Madney · M. E. Abdelrahim (✉) · H. Saeed
Clinical Pharmacy Department, Faculty of Pharmacy, Beni-suef University, Beni-suef, Egypt

© The Editor(s) (if applicable) and The Author(s), under exclusive license to Springer Nature Switzerland AG 2020
N. Vargas, A. M. Esquinas (eds.), *Covid-19 Airway Management and Ventilation Strategy for Critically Ill Older Patients*, https://doi.org/10.1007/978-3-030-55621-1_18

Table 18.1 Protective strategies to avoid aerosolization

1. Helmet interface covering the entire patient head
2. Total facemasks or oronasal masks with vent holes or with filter is placed between the mask and vent valve to minimize the spread of the virus
3. Rooms with adequate natural ventilation of at least 160 L/s airflow for a patient
4. Rooms with negative pressure in which the direction of the airflow is controlled and the air is changed at least 12 times/h
5. Protective equipment (PPE) as particulate respirators, eye protection, and gloves
6. Applying profound paralysis before instrumental airway

the helmet interface is not routinely used in clinical practice and its resources are limited. The alternative options are total facemasks (TFM) or conventional oronasal (NO) masks but masks with vent holes are preferred to be avoided unless a filter is placed between the mask and vent valve to minimize the spread of the virus [5]. Viral filters can filter aerosolized respiratory secretions that potentially contain the virus, rather than the ability to filter the virus itself [1]. Several precautions should be taken during HFNC and NIV procedures. They should be performed in rooms with adequate natural ventilation of at least 160 L/s airflow for a patient or in rooms with negative pressure in which the direction of the airflow is controlled and the air is changed at least 12 times/h. Preferably, the patient is placed in a single room where the number of persons in the room is limited to the minimum required to care for the patient. Additionally, HCWs should use personal protective equipment (PPE) as particulate respirators, eye protection, and gloves [8]. HCWs should ensure profound paralysis before instrumenting the airway with adequate dose and time for effect. ETO_2 monitoring is needed to minimize duration for which face mask is applied by identifying the earliest occurrence of adequate pre-oxygenation. Required ventilation pressures should be minimized by using neuromuscular blockade, 45° head elevation, and an oropharyngeal airway. Finally, the high gas flow should be avoided if no indication as the dispersal of liquid at 60 L/min is minimal and significantly less than that caused by coughing and sneezing, providing that nasal cannulae are well fitted [9, 10].

18.3 Conclusion

Aerosol-generating procedures carry a potential increased risk of nosocomial infection to healthcare workers with COVID-19 which necessities application of many protective strategies including using helmet interface, total face masks or conventional oronasal masks with vent holes secured with viral filters, ensuring adequate natural ventilation or applying profound paralysis before instrumental airway, wearing personal protective equipment by healthcare workers, minimizing ventilation pressures and avoiding high flow if no indication.

References

1. Brewster DJ, et al. Consensus statement: safe airway society principles of airway management and tracheal intubation specific to the COVID-19 adult patient group. Med J Aust. 2020;212(10):1.
2. Harb HS, et al. Performance of large spacer versus nebulizer T-piece in single-limb noninvasive ventilation. Respir Care. 2018;63(11):1360–9.
3. Casanova LM, et al. Effects of air temperature and relative humidity on coronavirus survival on surfaces. Appl Environ Microbiol. 2010;76(9):2712–7.
4. van Doremalen N, et al. Aerosol and surface stability of SARS-CoV-2 as compared with SARS-CoV-1. N Engl J Med. 2020;382:1564–7.
5. Guan L, et al. More awareness is needed for severe acute respiratory syndrome coronavirus 2019 transmission through exhaled air during non-invasive respiratory support: experience from China. Eur Respir J. 2020;55(3):2000352.
6. Parodi SM, Liu VX. From containment to mitigation of COVID-19 in the US. JAMA. 2020;323:1441.
7. Rodriguez AME, et al. Clinical review: helmet and non-invasive mechanical ventilation in critically ill patients. Crit Care. 2013;17(2):223.
8. World Health Organization. Infection prevention and control during health care when novel coronavirus (nCoV) infection is suspected: interim guidance, January 2020. Geneva: World Health Organization; 2020.
9. Hui DS, et al. Exhaled air dispersion during high-flow nasal cannula therapy versus CPAP via different masks. Eur Respir J. 2019;53(4):1802339.
10. Kotoda M, et al. Assessment of the potential for pathogen dispersal during high-flow nasal therapy. J Hosp Infect. 2019;104(4):534–7.

Part V

The Setting

The Older Patients in Subacute Units

19

Alonso Peinado Cano

19.1 Introduction

The coronavirus disease COVID-19 (SARS-CoV-2) is an infection disease that mainly affects the respiratory system, with the manifestation of interstitial pneumonia and severe acute respiratory syndrome [1]. The team of medical doctors that is primarily involved has been composed of infectious disease specialist, pneumologist, and anesthesiologists. Although no age group is safe from the SARS-CoV-2 infection, the burden is higher and severe for persons aged 70 years and over, with documented mortality rates of more than 20% among octogenarians [2]. It is clear that the COVID-19-susceptible population involves older people and people with certain underlying medical conditions (such as cardiovascular diseases, diabetes mellitus, renal failure, respiratory diseases), which requires more attention and care [3].

This sudden health emergency severely challenged the World Health System, in particular acute care hospital and intensive care units. In many hospital, geriatric observation units were created, the experience of which can be extremely useful for European countries, the Unites State, and all countries that in the coming days will face a similar situation. The presence of multiple pre-exiting comorbidities is correlated with more severe COVID-19 infection, causing a geriatric emergency worldwide and reflecting the presence of pre-existing physical and/or cognitive fragility [4].

Along with the outbreak of the epidemic of 2019 novel coronavirus, the number of older patient infected with COVID-19 was increasing in the world and it brought a serious threat to life and health.

M.D. in 061-EPES (Company publishes health emergencies). Almería, Spain. NIMV expert by *International School* of Non Invasive Mechanical Ventilation.

A. P. Cano (✉)
Department of Intermediate Care, Virgen del Mar-Vithas Hospital, Almería, Spain

N. Vargas, A. M. Esquinas (eds.), *Covid-19 Airway Management and Ventilation Strategy for Critically Ill Older Patients*, https://doi.org/10.1007/978-3-030-55621-1_19

173

A study in the New England Journal of Medicine (NEJM) by Guan reported the clinical characteristic of coronavirus diseases 2019 in China that the rate of older patients older than 65 years with COVID-19 was 15.1%.

It was probed that population including old people was generally susceptible, and the older patients with high infection rate and fatality (Yang, Yu et al. 2020). As a new disease and a new global health issue, COVID-19 infection is understandable that it causes anxiety and fear among the older population, due to its high spread. In addition, aging population has been one of the largest problems in many countries, and there were a higher prevalence of multimorbidity and lower resistance in older patients (Feng, Liu, Guan, and Moor 2012; Low et al. 2019), no doubt, there are many old people who will face the risk of infected with COVID-19 with the globalization and aging population. The risk of having an aging and infected elderly population imposes a heavy burden to healthcare systems in the world [5].

19.2   General Remarks

Results of a recent selected cohort analysis of 1099 patients of COVID-19 across China have shown that up to 15% (173/1099) developed severe disease according to the clinical criteria of severe community pneumonia of the American Thoracic Society [6]. Of these, 19% entered in intensive care units, requiring the use of mechanical ventilation, both invasive and noninvasive. In addition, 2.9% (5/173) required extracorporeal oxygenation systems. A recent publication with 191 patients COVID-19 infected admitted to hospitals in Wuhan gives 31% patients with ARDS with a mortality of 93% [7]. For this reason, adequate and staggered therapy is important for COVID-19 patients, regardless of their age.

The combination of advanced age and invasive ventilation were associated with increased hospital mortality. This ratio seems to increase as age increases [8]. However age should not imply restrictions in medical care. Because it does not constitute an independent mortality factor. High mortality, frequent comorbidities, and overall functional loss make bioethical considerations of paramount importance in decision-making in elderly patients with acute respiratory failure [9].

In the individual assessment of the patient, we must take into account their functional state, underlying diseases, and quality of life, respecting the decisions made by the patient. In hospitalized elderly patients and in situations of hypoxemic, hypercapnic respiratory failure, or both, NIV may be a well-tolerated as well as beneficial strategy, besides, it produces clinical and blood gases improvement of the patients. NIV reduces hospital stay, the need for endotracheal intubation, the incidence of pneumonia associated with mechanical ventilation, and even mortality.

Patients in whom an order not to intubate is established, either due to their advanced age or their terminal situation, NIV represents an optimal and sometimes unique strategy for the treatment of ARF [10]. It may be appropriate to reverse the situation of acute respiratory failure, as a comfort measure, or to delay death in a terminal situation, sometimes it may be necessary [9, 11].

Despite the disadvantages, advanced age constitutes a risk factor for poor response to NIV. This may be due to greater severity of pathologies and cognitive decline, more frequently in this age group [12]. NIV reduces the need for sedation and relaxation, which prevents associated long-term problems such as myopathies and muscle atrophies, frequent in patients undergoing MV in critical care units. Sedation may be necessary when starting NIV, due to a certain degree of anxiety, which usually disappears with adaptation to the technique and clinical improvement.

One of the most important factors to obtain good results with the use of noninvasive ventilation does not depend on the patients, but on the health personnel who manage it, who must be well trained. Having experienced staff in this type of techniques also makes it possible to apply them outside intensive care units, being of vital importance in elderly and terminally ill patients.

NIV can be used intermittently, allowing the patient to speak taking part in clinical decisions. They also allow the patient to eat and drink. The maintenance of these functions seems to represent important factors in the recovery of this type of patients [13].

In general, tolerance to NIMV in elderly patients is good and reduces mortality, the need for intubation, and the risk of associated complications. It can represent the therapeutic ceiling in specifying elderly patients [9].

Isolation measures are essential for patients suspected or COVID-19 infected, avoiding contagion with other patients and health personnel. The availability of personal protective equipment must be guaranteed to treat these patients.

19.3 Methods

Given the resources we have in the current pandemic, we need to anticipate the scenarios, adjusting resources rationally. Be prepared and work together to overcome the epidemic. In the subacute units we must identify patients with ARF susceptible to HFNO and noninvasive ventilation and be prepared to make the switch to invasive ventilation if appropriate[14].

I find monitoring essential in the management of respiratory failure caused by COVID. These patients should be placed in an individual room, ideally with negative pressure and centralized monitoring (pulse oximetry, heart rate) with video surveillance [14] if possible. When resources are depleted, we will maintain a minimum distance of 2 m between patients and the area will be considered a dirty area.

19.3.1 Therapeutic Respiratory in Subacute Units for Old Patients

In SARS-CoV-2 infection, like other processes that cause respiratory failure, the respiratory strategy proposed by Scala and Heunks can be used. The base of the therapeutic pyramid consists of oxygen supply in different concentration, finding several therapeutic steps:

First Step: Standard oxygen therapy.

Oxygen with reservoir bag (10–15 L/min) to keep $SpO_2 > 92$–93% and they need prone position to reach that oximetry [15].

Older patients usually present cardiac and pulmonary comorbidities; therefore they require surveillance. Some end up being candidates for HFNO or NIVM, requiring close surveillance in subacute units, under continuous monitoring.

Second Step: High-flow nasal oxygen (HFNO). Should be used in selected patient with hypoxemic respiratory failure.

In general, HFNO is a valid option for standard oxygen therapy. Adult HFNO system can deliver 60 L/min of gas flow and FiO_2 up to 1.0; the gas must be hot and 100% humidified. The advantages with respect to conventional oxygen are a constant contribution of FiO_2, reduction of dead space, and the generation of a positive pressure (intravascular fluid redistribution and alveolar recruitment).

Compared with standard oxygen therapy, HFNO reduces the need for intubation. Patients with hypercapnia (exacerbation of obstructive lung diseases, cardiogenic pulmonary edema), hemodynamic instability, multiorgan failure, or abnormal mental status should generally not receive HFNO. However, emerging data suggest that HFNO may be safe in patients with mild-moderate and non-worsening hypercapnia.

Patients receiving HFNO should be in a monitored setting and cared for by experienced personnel capable of endotracheal intubation in case the patient acutely deteriorates or does not improve after a short trial [15, 16].

Third Step: NIMV/CPAP.

For the use of noninvasive therapy we recommend the following considerations:

1. Lung protection therapy: High PEEP (10–14 cmH$_2$O), VT 6 mL/kg, PS (pressure support) no more than 5 cmH$_2$O.
2. Interface rotation. Hypoxemic patients do not tolerate periods without noninvasive therapy due to alveolar recruitment and early hypoxia. We recommend alternating NIV/CPAP with HFNO continuously, minimizing side effects. We must evaluate interface rotation each 6–8 h.

We recommend the use of helmet or total face interface; the use of orofacial interface may be accepted. Physicians did not use the nasal interface in acute patients with hypoxemic failure respiratory secondary to respiratory infection because of more aerosols.

These interfaces can be used as long as safety standards are met, since noninvasive ventilation is considered a dispersal mechanism for aerosols [17].

We use noninvasive ventilation in subacute units in the following cases:

- As initial therapy in selected cases, treated by NIV experts and with safe conditions for the patient, including elderly patients.
- As bridging therapy until the start of invasive ventilation if appropriate.
- As the only therapy when an invasive ventilation respirator is not available.
- For the medical transport of patients.
- As palliative therapy in selected cases.
- In weaning phase of invasive ventilation.
- In patient with order not to intubate.
- In very old patients, over 85 years.

Patients undergoing invasive mechanical ventilation or who require ECMO will be placed in trained units.

19.3.2 Prone Position

Noninvasive ventilation considerations in the prone position for old patients in subacute units:

NI strategy in prone position (CPAP/NIV/HFNO) can be useful in selected cases. There are a few studies on the effect of prone position in patients under NIV and severe hypoxemia, but it seems that it may be a strategy to consider in an early stage and in select patient. We understand that using the prone position can imply an unacceptable burden of care in certain circumstances and must be done if safety measure for heath personnel and patients can be maintained. In case of opting for a prone position strategy, the recommendations are the following:

- Start of NIV in supine position and respiratory stabilization.
- Prone test in both (NIV/CPAP) during 30 min.
- Hold until signs of tiredness appear or the patient is not comfortable.
- Try to pronate the patient at least twice a day [17, 18].

19.3.3 Drugs

We usually use pharmacological measure for adaptation and comfort to NIV therapy. Often our elderly patients are agitated due to hypoxia and their underlying diseases.

These are measures aimed at controlling tachypnea and increasing comfort and adherence to the treatment of patients. The primary goal is to decrease dyspnea. The secondary objective is the initial decrease in respiratory rate to facilitate adaptation NIV.

Pharmacological measures depend on the experience of the physician and the safety and monitoring environment. The administration of drug should always be IV in a titrated and progressive way until evaluation of the effects. In any cases, these recommendations can be adapted in relation to the protocols of superficial sedation and pharmacological control of dyspnea.

- Initial drug: Morphine in boluses titrated at 3 mg, with a latency between 20–30 min for repeating doses.
- Second-line drugs. Remifentanil, dexmedetomidine in continuous perfusion, always in controlled monitoring environments and managed by expert personnel.
- Third-line drugs: Propofol in continuous perfusion, always in controlled monitoring environments and managed by expert personnel [17].

19.3.4 Recommendation on Safety and Environments Health for the Prevention of Contagion

Health personnel who attend cases under investigation or confirmed for COVID-19 infection under treatment with NIV therapy must wear personal protective equipment for the prevention of infection. Aerosol generation procedures have been associated with an increased risk of transmission of airborne pathogens. Preventive measures must be directed to droplet-borne microorganisms and contact [14]:

- FFP2 mask or preferably FFP3 if available.
- Protective glasses with integral frame.
- Collect long hair in a ponytail or low bun inside a surgical cap.
- Gloves.
- Waterproof microbiological protection gowns of long sleeve.

However, if the technique fails and we must proceed to an endotracheal intubation, we will need a more secure protective equipment.

The location of the patients in the hospital setting is related to the possibility of carrying aerosol-generating operations. In this sense, the patients with severe hypoxemia would be admitted to the special units.

For intrahospital transfer, the patients and the professional transferring the patient will wear a surgical mask. During the transfer, the patient's bed will be covered with a clean disposable sheet that will be eliminated as group III residue.

Although al the present time there doubts regarding with dispersion of particles in the COVID-19, in the SARS epidemic some articles were published, it showed the distribution of particles with the NIV of a single circuit and exhalation port of more than 4 ft. (1, 25 m).

Preferably use double-branch configuration, since they provide hermeticism to the respiratory circuit, both inspiratory and expiratory. High-efficiency antimicrobial filters should be placed in the expiratory branch to avoid contamination from the patients to respirator. In case of not having double-branch system and having to use the simple branch, you should locate the expiratory orphic in the single socket and place a high efficiency and low antimicrobial filter resistance to minimize dispersion of exhaled gas, which can pollute the ambient air. It seems feasible, likewise, to interpose a T-piece in the circuit to fit the filter and the intentional leak; even the increase in the dead space must be taken into account. In the event that a high efficiency antimicrobial filter cannot be applied to the expiratory orifice, a high-efficiency antimicrobial filter is placed between the interface of the patient (no expiratory holes)/ventilator and the circuit. In this case, a higher resistance may require modifying the fan parameters to increase the support pressure level.

A feasible alternative to double-branch system or one branch with leakage is the use of single-branch systems with active valve and antimicrobial filter placement at an active valve outlet.

I do not recommend using heat and moisture exchangers (HME).

I recommend using an elbow without an anti-asphyxia valve; this forces us to take extreme care of the patient, in the event of possible failure of the ventilation equipment.

Consider that these patients are located in highly complex rooms, under the continuous care of expert healthcare personnel. Therefore accidental disconnection not detected or corrected in time is unlikely, provided there is a safe nursing staff ratio. We discourage the use of anti-rebreathing elbow (which is also houses an anti-asphyxia valve) due to the risk of greater dispersion of expired air [14].

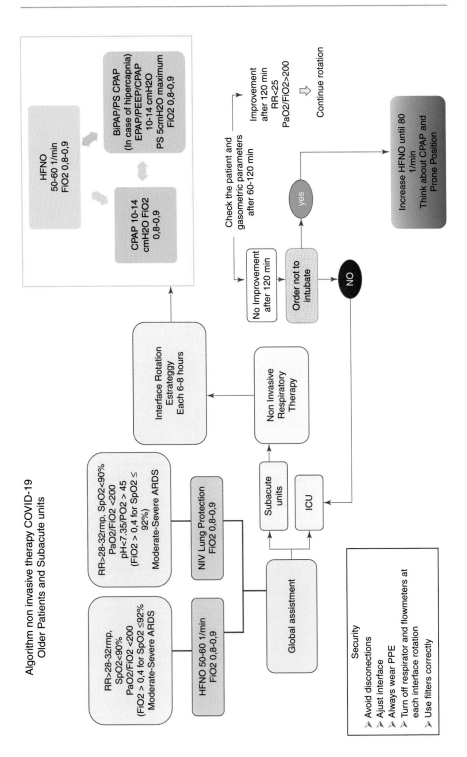

Algorithm non invasive therapy COVID-19
Older Patients and Subacute units

19.4 Conclusion

1. Elderly patients confirmed or suspected of COVID-19 infection have a high proportion of severe cases. COVID-19 infection is susceptible to a relatively high mortality rate in the elderly population. We should pay more attention to older patients.
2. Tolerance to NIMV in elderly patients is good and reduces mortality, the need for intubation, and the risk of associated complications. It can represent the therapeutic ceiling in specifying elderly patients. NIV reduces hospital stay and the need for endotracheal intubation.
3. Having experienced staff in NIV also makes it possible to apply them outside intensive care units, being of vital importance in elderly and terminally ill patients.
4. Isolation measures are essential for patients suspected or COVID-19 infected. Avoiding contagion with other patients and health personnel. The availability of Personal Protective Equipment must be guaranteed to treat these patients.
5. From an ethical point of view, we cannot abandon any patient and we must cure or alleviate their illness, reaching a worthy therapeutic ceiling if necessary. Involves caregivers and family members in decision-making and goal-setting throughout the management of ARF-COVID-19.

References

1. Jordan RE, Adab P, Cheng KK. Covid-19: risk factors for severe disease and death. BMJ. 2020;368:m1198.
2. Livingston E, Bucher K. Coronavirus disease 2019 (COVID-19) in Italy. JAMA. 2020;323:1335. https://doi.org/10.1001/jama.2020.4344.
3. Yang J, Zheng Y, Gou X, et al. Prevalence of comorbilities in the novel Wuhan coronavirus (COVID-19) infection: a systematic review and meta-analysis. Int J Infect Dis. 2020;94:91–5. https://doi.org/10.1016/j.ijd.2020.03.01732173574.
4. Gemelli Against COVID-19 Geriatrics Team, Landi F, Barillaro C, Bellini A, Brandi V, Carfi A, Ciprinai C, D'Angelo E, Falsiroli C, Fusco D, Landi G, Liperoti R, Lo Monaco M, Martone A, Marzetti E, Pagano F, Pais C, Russo A, Salini S, Tosato M, Tummolo A, Benvenuto Zuccala G, Bernabei R. The geriatrician: the frontline specialist in the treatment of COVID-19 patients. J Am Med Assoc. 2020; https://doi.org/10.1016/j.jamada.2020.04.017.
5. Niu S, Tian S, Jung L, Kang X, Zhang L, Lian H, Zhang J. Beijing Emergency Medical Center. Clinical characteristics of older patients infected With COVID-19: a descriptive study. Arch Gerontol Geriatr. 2020;89:104058.
6. Guan W, Ni Z, Hu Y, Liang W, et al. Clinical characteristics of coronavirus disease 2019 in China. N Engl J Med. 2020;382:1708. https://doi.org/10.1056/NEJMoa2002032.
7. Zhou F, Yu T, Du R, et al. Clinical course and risk factors for mortality of adult inpatients with COVID-19 in Wuhan, China: a retrospective cohort study. Lancet. 2020;395:P1054–62. https://doi.org/10.1016/S0140-6736(20)30566-3.
8. Farfel JM, Franca SA, Sitta MC. Age, invasive ventilatory support and outcomes in elderly patients admitted to intensive care units. Age Ageing. 2009;38:515–20.
9. Fundamentos de Metodología y organización hospitalaria en Ventilación Mecánica No Invasiva: Antonio M. Esquinas, July 2014. Ventilación Mecánica no Invasiva en Geriatría:

Pedro Cuesta Santos, Pilar Aguirre Puig, María del Cielo Canitrot Janeiro, María de los Angeles Orallo Morán.

10. Sacarpazza P, Incorvaia C. Effect of non-invasive mechanical ventilation in elderly patients with hypercapnia acute-on-chronic respiratory failure and do-not-intubate order. Int J COPD. 2008;3(4):797–801.
11. Kacmarek RM. Should noninvasive ventilation be used with the do-not-intubate patient? Respir Care. 2009;54(2):223–9; discussion 229–31.
12. Brochard L. Mechanical ventilation. Invasive versus non invasive. Eur Respir J. 2003;22(Suppl. 47):31s–7s.
13. Cannolly MJ. Non invasive ventilation in elderly patientes with acute exacerbation of COPD: bringing pressure to bear. Age Ageing. 2006;35:1–2.
14. Cinesi Gómez C, et al. Recomendaciones de consenso respecto al soporte respiratorio no invasivo en el paciente adulto con insuficiencia respiratoria aguda secundaria a infección por SARS-CoV-2. Rev Esp Anestesiol Reanim. 2020;67:261. https://doi.org/10.1016/j.redar.2020.03.006.
15. Clinical management of severe acute respiratory infection (SARI) when COVID-19 disease is suspected. WHO (World Health Organization). Interim guidance, 13 March 2020.
16. Rpchwerg B, Brochard L, Elliot MV, Hess D, Hill NS, Nava S, et al. Official ERS/ATS clinical practice guidelines: noninvasive ventilation for acute respiratory failure. Eur Respir J. 2017;50(2):1602426. https://doi.org/10.1183/13993003.02426-2016.
17. Recomendaciones para el uso de Ventilación Mecánica no Invasiva, sistemas CPAP no mecánicos y Terapia de alto Flujo en pacientes con infección respiratoria por COVID-19. Grupo Multidisciplinar Español de Expertos en Terapias Respiratorias No Invasivas-VMNI-CR Group. Alonso, J.M. and Cols et al March 2020.
18. Lin Ding L, Wang L, Ma W, He H. Efficacy and safety of early prono positioning combined with HFNC or NIV in moderate to severe ARDS: a multi-center prospective cohort study. Crit Care. 2020;24:28. https://doi.org/10.1186/s13054-020-2738-5.

The ICU

20

Sven Stieglitz

Abbreviations

ECMO   Extracorporeal membrane oxygenation
HFNC   High-flow nasal cannula
ICU   Intensive care unit
NIV   Noninvasive ventilation

20.1 The ICU

20.1.1 Introduction

Elderly population is defined as people aged 65 and over in contrast to working age (15–64 age). The definition for elderly patients is not necessarily consistent with the definition for geriatric patients since aging is an individual process [1]. Therefore, the typical trials of frailty, comorbidities, and disability are better characterizing geriatric patients [2]. Another important characteristic of geriatric patients is the development of dementia. Almost 15% of individuals older than 70 years have dementia [3]. Polymorbidity leads to polypharmacy which may cause problems as an increasing number of drug prescriptions is increasing the risk of adverse drug events which is clearly correlated to old age [4].

S. Stieglitz (✉)
Department of Pneumology, Allergy, Sleep and Intensive Care Medicine, Petrus Hospital Wuppertal, Wuppertal, Germany
e-mail: Sven.stieglitz@cellitinnen.de

© The Editor(s) (if applicable) and The Author(s), under exclusive license to
Springer Nature Switzerland AG 2020
N. Vargas, A. M. Esquinas (eds.), *Covid-19 Airway Management and Ventilation Strategy for Critically Ill Older Patients*, https://doi.org/10.1007/978-3-030-55621-1_20

183

Table 20.1 Prevention and treatment of delirium is essential in the old and very old patients at ICU

Prevention and treatment of delirium at ICU	
Maintenance of day-night rhythm	Darken the room at night
	Avoid nursing or other interventions at night
	Turn off the alarming in the patients' room at night
Family caregiving	Allow visitation of patients
	Allow touching of the patients by relatives
Promote mobility	Physiotherapists
	Verticalization of the patients whenever possible
	No fixation or medical sedation
Relaxing music and smells (aromatherapy)	During daytime

It correlates with mortality as well with cognitive impairment and functional status after treatment

It is estimated that 20% of hospitalized patients over age 65 suffer from delirium [5] which is associated in an elderly patient with an additional burden, a possible loss of potential for rehabilitation, and a marked increase in mortality. An appropriate tool for assessment of delirium on intensive care unit (ICU) is the CAM-ICU [6]. Non-pharmacological treatments include the creation of a calm and patient-centered environment, promotion of mobility, optimal level of stimulation with fixed day/night rhythm, and the involvement of relatives [7] (Table 20.1). Taking these factors into account, it is obvious that the ICU environment is unfavorable regarding prevention and treatment of delirium.

Demographic data of OECD indicate that in economically developed countries the proportion of elderly persons was increasing constantly over the past 30 years and varies now between 16% (USA) and 23% (Italy). As the population ages, the number of older patients treated at ICU also increases. Between 2001 and 2008, 45.7% of the patients were aged above 60, therefrom 41% were aged 75–84 and 23% were aged 85 and above [8]. The in-hospital mortality was 19% in the age group 65–74 and 28% in the group over 84. Especially in the elderly, the focus on treatment is not only mortality but also on maintaining function, especially mobility and cognitive function.

Epidemiology studies show that morbidity and mortality of COVID-19 increases at an age above 65 [9]. Mortality of patients at an age above 80 is more than 15% [10]. Therefore, COVID-19 is a disease of the elderly with severe respiratory complications where the need for ICU treatment has to be evaluated early in the course of the disease.

20.1.2 What Is an Intensive Care Unit?

An ICU is based in a defined geographic area of a hospital that provides life-preserving measures in acute medicine. The treatment of the patients is usually provided by a defined multidisciplinary team of critical care nurses and intensivists that are supported by respiratory therapists and other valuable doctors. Some medical measures are characteristic for ICU as, for example, medical and technical support of circulation and mechanical ventilation though the introduction of noninvasive ventilation offered the opportunity for mechanical ventilation outside of an ICU under certain circumstances.

The task force of the World Federation of Societies of Intensive and Critical Care Medicine distinguishes between different levels of ICU [11]: - a level 1 ICU is above all capable of providing; - a level 2 ICU can provide invasive monitoring in combination with short time basic life support and it needs a level 3 ICU for the full spectru of monitoring and life support technologies. Level 3 ICU is put on the same level as ICU in general. In pandemics as SARS-CoV2, ICU beds are a precious resource. On the other hand, several studies suggest that less ICU use would not worsen patient outcomes, especially when patients with low-mortality conditions are treated [12]. Therefore, improving ICU triage practices is important not only from a medical point of view but also to limit the expansion of intensive care costs.

20.1.3 Needs of Elderly Patients with SARS-CoV2 at ICU

In general, partial support or complete substitution of ventilation has made tremendous progress in the recent years. On the one end of the spectrum there is the expensive and invasive use of extracorporeal devices (ECMO) although a clear benefit in concern of mortality in clinical studies have not been shown yet; on the other end there is the introduction of high-flow-systems (high-flow nasal cannula, HFNC), which uses a high flow of mixed gas concentrations (humidified, heated air with defined levels of oxygen), noninvasive ventilation (ventilation with mask interfaces), or continuous positive airway pressure (CPAP). The combination of prone position with invasive ventilation has been demonstrated to improve oxygenation and mortality [13]. The next step was the introduction of early prone position in combination with HFNC and NIV [14, 15] which is able to improve oxygenation [16].

In COVID-19 the extent of hypoxemia often exaggerates the extent of radiological findings. Therefore, next to anatomical changes (alveolar filling, microembolism) a functional component is an important factor. It is discussed that the hypoxic pulmonary vasoconstriction (Euler-Liljestrand mechanism) is attenuated, which then leads to an increase of ventilation-perfusion inequality. Sedation and relaxation of the patients in the context of invasive ventilation aggravates this mismatch often leading to severe hypoxemia despite intubation.

The most important risk factors of mortality for very elderly patients at ICU are the use of inotropes and severity of illness [17]. Since the usage of inotrope should be avoided, also sedation and invasive ventilation should be avoided. Therefore, ICU treating elderly patients with severe hypoxemia like patients with COVID-19 should be able to offer treatment options like CPAP/NIV and HFNC in combination with prone or lateral position with high quality. The recommended level of experience usually requires the support by a pneumologist and respiratory therapist. In a pandemic scenario the availability of ECMO is less important.

Table 20.2 SOFA and CRB-65 are well introduced and may be used also in COVID-19

Suitable assessment at ICU for elderly patients	
Assessment of acute situation	SOFA CRB-65
Frailty	Rockwood Clinical Frailty Scale [19]
Comorbidities	Charlson comorbidity index [20]
Polypharmacy	Identify anticholinergic burden [21] Identify drug interactions
Malnutrition	Albumin serum concentration Body mass index BMI
Cognitive impairment	Mini-Mental State Examination MMST
Delirium	CAM-ICU [6]
Activities of daily live	ADL scale [22] IADL [23]

The geriatric assessment listed helps to characterize elderly patients at ICU

The old and very old patients are characterized by frailty, comorbidities, polypharmacy, malnutrition, cognitive impairment, delirium, and reduced activities of daily life. Several instruments and assessments exist to characterize these patients properly (Table 20.2).

20.1.4 Structural Needs of an ICU Treating COVID-19 Patients

Quarantine and isolation of patients with COVID-19 is necessary. Cohorting of infectious patients is possible but it has to be ensured that there is no concomitant infection with other pathogens like influenza. Ideally, a limited team of doctors and nurses are caring exclusively for the COVID-19 patients. The presence of unnecessary staff in the room must be avoided.

The ideal structure of an ICU contains negative pressure rooms. The negative pressure helps preventing the spread of contagious aerosol into the ICU and other hospital facilities. It is recommended to perform aerosol-generating procedures like tracheal intubation, bronchoscopies, or noninvasive positive pressure ventilation within this room. This lowers the risk of cross-contamination among the ICU and infection for the staff and patients outside the room without influencing the risk for the staff working in this room [18]. Due to costs, negative pressure rooms are only available in few ICUs and those ICUs equipped with negative pressure rooms usually have few negative pressure rooms. The most important sources of infection are aerosols and microaerosols. These aerosols may stay within the room for 20–30 min. Healthcare staff working within the patient room should wear fitted respirators masks next to other personal protective equipment (e.g., eye protection). Keeping distance (1.5 m) and airing the rooms extensively (windows open for 15 min every hour) are essential for protection of the medical staff.

Concerning prophylaxis and treatment of delirium (Table 20.1) the structure of an ICU is usually not ideal. In this regard, treating COVID-19 is an even greater challenge since many of the ideas are difficult to realize. Social distancing and isolation of the patients aggravates these problems and promotes the development of delirium furthermore. Therefore it is essential to end the isolation of a COVID-19 patient when he is no longer contagious. This is important not only with regard to delirium but also to discharge the professional staff as well as economic costs.

References

1. Boyd CM, Ritchie CS, Tipton EF, Studenski SA, Wieland D. From bedside to bench: summary from the American Geriatrics Society/National Institute on Aging Research conference on comorbidity and multiple morbidity in older adults. Aging Clin Exp Res. 2008;20(3):181–8. https://doi.org/10.1007/BF03324775.
2. Fried LP, Tangen CM, Walston J, Newman AB, Hirsch C, Gottdiener J, Seeman T, Tracy R, Kop WJ, Burke G, McBurnie MA, Cardiovascular Health Study Collaborative Research G. Frailty in older adults: evidence for a phenotype. J Gerontol A Biol Sci Med Sci. 2001;56(3):M146–56.
3. Whitson HE, Cronin-Golomb A, Cruickshanks KJ, Gilmore GC, Owsley C, Peelle JE, Recanzone G, Sharma A, Swenor B, Yaffe K, Lin FR. American Geriatrics Society and National Institute on Aging bench-to-bedside conference: sensory impairment and cognitive decline in older adults. J Am Geriatr Soc. 2018;66(11):2052–8. https://doi.org/10.1111/jgs.15506.
4. Mangin D, Bahat G, Golomb BA, Mallery LH, Moorhouse P, Onder G, Petrovic M, Garfinkel D. International group for reducing inappropriate medication use & polypharmacy (IGRIMUP): position statement and 10 recommendations for action. Drugs Aging. 2018;35(7):575–87. https://doi.org/10.1007/s40266-018-0554-2.
5. Inouye SK, Bogardus ST Jr, Charpentier PA, Leo-Summers L, Acampora D, Holford TR, Cooney LM Jr. A multicomponent intervention to prevent delirium in hospitalized older patients. N Engl J Med. 1999;340(9):669–76. https://doi.org/10.1056/NEJM199903043400901.
6. Gusmao-Flores D, Salluh JI, Chalhub RA, Quarantini LC. The confusion assessment method for the intensive care unit (CAM-ICU) and intensive care delirium screening checklist (ICDSC) for the diagnosis of delirium: a systematic review and meta-analysis of clinical studies. Crit Care. 2012;16(4):R115. https://doi.org/10.1186/cc11407.
7. Lorenzl S, Fusgen I, Noachtar S. Acute confusional states in the elderly—diagnosis and treatment. Dtsch Arztebl Int. 2012;109(21):391–9; quiz 400. https://doi.org/10.3238/arztebl.2012.0391.
8. Fuchs L, Chronaki CE, Park S, Novack V, Baumfeld Y, Scott D, McLennan S, Talmor D, Celi L. ICU admission characteristics and mortality rates among elderly and very elderly patients. Intensive Care Med. 2012;38(10):1654–61. https://doi.org/10.1007/s00134-012-2629-6.
9. Zhu N, Zhang D, Wang W, Li X, Yang B, Song J, Zhao X, Huang B, Shi W, Lu R, Niu P, Zhan F, Ma X, Wang D, Xu W, Wu G, Gao GF, Tan W, China Novel Coronavirus I, Research T. A Novel Coronavirus from patients with pneumonia in China, 2019. N Engl J Med. 2020;382(8):727–33. https://doi.org/10.1056/NEJMoa2001017.
10. Zhou F, Yu T, Du R, Fan G, Liu Y, Liu Z, Xiang J, Wang Y, Song B, Gu X, Guan L, Wei Y, Li H, Wu X, Xu J, Tu S, Zhang Y, Chen H, Cao B. Clinical course and risk factors for mortality of adult inpatients with COVID-19 in Wuhan, China: a retrospective cohort study. Lancet. 2020;395(10229):1054–62. https://doi.org/10.1016/S0140-6736(20)30566-3.
11. Marshall JC, Bosco L, Adhikari NK, Connolly B, Diaz JV, Dorman T, Fowler RA, Meyfroidt G, Nakagawa S, Pelosi P, Vincent JL, Vollman K, Zimmerman J. What is an intensive care unit? A report of the task force of the world Federation of Societies of intensive and critical care medicine. J Crit Care. 2017;37:270–6. https://doi.org/10.1016/j.jcrc.2016.07.015.
12. Valley TS, Noritomi DT. ICU beds: less is more? Yes. Intensive Care Med. 2020;25:1–3. https://doi.org/10.1007/s00134-020-06042-1.

13. Scholten EL, Beitler JR, Prisk GK, Malhotra A. Treatment of ARDS with prone positioning. Chest. 2017;151(1):215–24. https://doi.org/10.1016/j.chest.2016.06.032.
14. Ding L, Wang L, Ma W, He H. Efficacy and safety of early prone positioning combined with HFNC or NIV in moderate to severe ARDS: a multi-center prospective cohort study. Crit Care. 2020;24(1):28. https://doi.org/10.1186/s13054-020-2738-5.
15. Feltracco P, Serra E, Barbieri S, Persona P, Rea F, Loy M, Ori C. Non-invasive ventilation in prone position for refractory hypoxemia after bilateral lung transplantation. Clin Transpl. 2009;23(5):748–50. https://doi.org/10.1111/j.1399-0012.2009.01050.x.
16. Stieglitz S, Frohnhofen H, Netzer N, Haidl P, Orth M, Schlesinger A. Recommendations for the treatment of elderly patients with COVID-19 from the taskforce for Gerontopneumology. Pneumologie. 2020; https://doi.org/10.1055/a-1177-3588.
17. Van Den Noortgate N, Vogelaers D, Afschrift M, Colardyn F. Intensive care for very elderly patients: outcome and risk factors for in-hospital mortality. Age Ageing. 1999;28(3):253–6. https://doi.org/10.1093/ageing/28.3.253.
18. Alhazzani W, Moller MH, Arabi YM, Loeb M, Gong MN, Fan E, Oczkowski S, Levy MM, Derde L, Dzierba A, Du B, Aboodi M, Wunsch H, Cecconi M, Koh Y, Chertow DS, Maitland K, Alshamsi F, Belley-Cote E, Greco M, Laundy M, Morgan JS, Kesecioglu J, McGeer A, Mermel L, Mammen MJ, Alexander PE, Arrington A, Centofanti JE, Citerio G, Baw B, Memish ZA, Hammond N, Hayden FG, Evans L, Rhodes A. Surviving Sepsis campaign: guidelines on the management of critically ill adults with Coronavirus disease 2019 (COVID-19). Intensive Care Med. 2020;46(5):854–87. https://doi.org/10.1007/s00134-020-06022-5.
19. Rockwood K, Song X, MacKnight C, Bergman H, Hogan DB, McDowell I, Mitnitski A. A global clinical measure of fitness and frailty in elderly people. CMAJ. 2005;173(5):489–95. https://doi.org/10.1503/cmaj.050051.
20. Charlson ME, Sax FL. The therapeutic efficacy of critical care units from two perspectives: a traditional cohort approach vs a new case-control methodology. J Chronic Dis. 1987;40(1):31–9. https://doi.org/10.1016/0021-9681(87)90094-4.
21. Salahudeen MS, Duffull SB, Nishtala PS. Anticholinergic burden quantified by anticholinergic risk scales and adverse outcomes in older people: a systematic review. BMC Geriatr. 2015;15:31. https://doi.org/10.1186/s12877-015-0029-9.
22. Katz S, Akpom CA. 12. Index of ADL. Med Care. 1976;14(5 Suppl):116–8. https://doi.org/10.1097/00005650-197605001-00018.
23. Lawton MP, Brody EM. Assessment of older people: self-maintaining and instrumental activities of daily living. Gerontologist. 1969;9(3):179–86.

The Admission of Older Patients with COVID-19 in the General Wards

21

Loredana Tibullo, Barbara Bonamassa, Attilio De Blasio, Daniela Verrillo, and Nicola Vargas

21.1 Introduction

Some criteria and selection tools are, in a general line, useful for recognition of all elderly patients with COVID-19 disease. Furthermore, many organisations may influence this criterion such as WHO, scientific medical society, a single government or health ministers and hospital management systems. In this chapter, we analysed the requirements for admission of the elderly patients in a general ward starting from triage evaluation using the new proposed tool for the selection. The necessity of a comprehensive geriatric assessment with a holistic vision has been not so crucial as in this period.

L. Tibullo (✉)
Medicine Department, Ward of Internal Medicine, San Giuseppe Moscati Hospital, Aversa, Italy

B. Bonamassa
Health Department, ASL NA2 North, Naples, Italy

A. De Blasio
Emergency Department, Maggiore Hospital, Parma, Italy

D. Verrillo · N. Vargas
Geriatric and Intensive Geriatric Cares, San Giuseppe Moscati Hospital, Avellino, Italy

© The Editor(s) (if applicable) and The Author(s), under exclusive license to Springer Nature Switzerland AG 2020
N. Vargas, A. M. Esquinas (eds.), *Covid-19 Airway Management and Ventilation Strategy for Critically Ill Older Patients*, https://doi.org/10.1007/978-3-030-55621-1_21

21.2 The Complexity of Older Patients

When screening suggests potential significant frailties in an older patient with COVID, the performance of comprehensive geriatric assessment (CGA) remains the optimal approach to identify risks better, and consequently appropriate treatment [1]. The holistic evaluation starts from the frailty and comorbidities and then from the medical history of the patient (Fig. 21.1). Older patients have often limited decisional capacity, and the assessment of their wishes and the possibility that a legal surrogate can decide on behalf of the patients is essential. The prognosis of older patients with COVID-19 is most unfavourable. The mortality rate is high. The possibility of an individual caring plan discussed by a multi-professional team and family members helps to manage these patients. The physicians are using some specific tools to evaluate the setting, and the prognosis also for older patients.

21.3 The Older with COVID-19 Recognition with a Score

In the presence of an older patient who needs hospitalisation, a comprehensive geriatric evaluation is mandatory. The decision-making process refers to, especially, the choice of an adequate setting. The necessity of interdisciplinary team may be

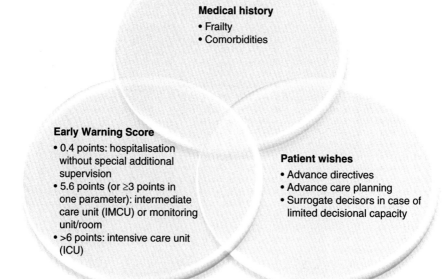

Fig. 21.1 Criteria for recognition of elderly patient with COVID-19

essential to evaluate the prognosis and reduce the emotional weight of the decision. Physicians use an evaluation of physiological parameter-based warning score to facilitate early recognition of patients with severe infection. Hospital admission is related to the severity classification. The score is a modified version of the National Early Warning Score (NEWS) (Fig. 21.2) with age ≥65 years added as an independent risk factor based on recent reports. According to the score assigned to the patient, we can have four categories: low, median, high, and exceptional [2, 3]. A special critical care team decides which patients need to be treated in the ICU, taking into consideration the disease severity, opportunity to benefit, and sources of support. The patient who shows a score of 0–4 points requires hospitalisation without special additional supervision. When the points are 5–6 (or ≥3 points in one

Early warning score for 2019-nCoV Infected Patients							
PARAMETERS	3	2	1	0	1	2	3
Age				<65			≥65
Respiration Rate	≤8		9 - 11	12 - 20		21 - 24	≥25
Oxygen Saturations	≤91	92 - 93	94 - 95	≥96			
Any Supplemental Oxygen		Yes		No			
Systolic BP	≤90	91 - 100	101 - 110	111- 219			≥220
Heart Rate	≤40		41 - 50	51 - 90	91 - 110	111 - 130	≥131
Consciousness				Alert			Drowsiness Letargy Coma Confusion
Temperature	≤35.0		35.1 - 36.0	36.1 - 38.0	38.1 - 39.0	≥39.1	

Early warning rules for 2019-nCoV Infected Patients					
Score	Risk Grading	Warning Level	Monitoring Frequency	Clinical Response	Solution
0	/		Q12h	Routine Monitoring	/
1 - 4	Low	Yellow	Q6h	Bedside evaluation by nurse	Maintain existing monitoring/ Increase monitoring frequency/ Inform doctor
5 - 6 or 3 in one parameter	Medium	Orange	Q1-2h	Bedside nurse notifies doctor for evaluation	Maintain existing treatment/ Adjust treatment plan/ CCRRT* remote consultation
≥7	High	Red	Continuous	Bedside nurse notifies doctor for emergency beside evaluation/ CCRRT remote consultation	CCRRT on site consultation
≥7	High	Black	Continuous	✓ Patients are extremely severe with irreversible end-stage diseases facing death, such as serious irreversible brain injury, irreversible multiple organ failure, end-stage chronic liver or lung disease, metastatic tumors, etc. ✓ Should be discussed urgently by the expert group about the admission decision.	

Fig. 21.2 Early Warning score for COVID-19 disease from Liao et al. [2]

parameter), an intermediate care unit (IMCU) or monitoring unit/room is necessary. If the patient reaches a score >6 points, the patient has to be admitted to the intensive care unit (ICU).

21.4 Clinical Evaluation and Risk Factors

Some investigations have identified the risk factors for the clinical outcomes of COVID-19 pneumonia. Older age was associated with greater risk of development of acute respiratory distress syndrome (ARDS) and death likely owing to less rigorous immune response. Although high fever was related to the development of ARDS, it was also associated with better outcomes among patients with ARDS. Other factors that may also help in the assessment of folder patients are: lymphopenia and neutropenia, lactate dehydrogenase (LDH) increase, increased D-dimers, and interleukin-6 [4]. Physicians who treated a patient who requires oxygen administration via nasal cannula/probe, Venturi mask or reservoir mask (max. 15 L/min, no nasal high-flow device) and continuous monitoring of vital parameters (SpO_2, blood pressure, heart rate and respiratory rate) is necessary admission in intermediate care or high dependency unit (HDU). For the patient who requires the use of high-flow oxygen therapy and non-invasive ventilation is not recommended the admission in the general wards and outside of an intensive care unit. Some critical risk discussed in other chapters of this book may influence the outcome, such as the risk of aerosols. In the case of rapid deterioration for the system failure, the possibility to admit the patient in an intensive care unit is an option that physicians have to provide. Hospital administrators, governments, and policy makers must work with ICU practitioners to prepare for a substantial increase in critical care bed capacity. They must protect healthcare workers from nosocomial transmission, physical exhaustion, and mental health issues that might be aggravated by the need to make ethically difficult decisions on the rationing of intensive care [5]. In the context of scarce ICU beds, alternative hospital admissions are necessary, and the organisation of high dependence units with the possibility of monitoring vital signs of older patients should be provided.

21.5 Conclusion

The selection of older patients with COVID disease includes the evaluation of many factors. Also, in this case, the CGS is the first step to assess the frailty. In light of the possible unfavourable outcome, it is necessary for the evaluation of the patient's wishes and the involvement of family members. The admission in the general wards has precise indications. Furthermore, the general ward may be an alternative in the case of the exclusion of older patients from ICU. The organisation of the general wards include the possibility of monitoring and a prompt admission in ICU if there is a rapid worsening of older patients' clinical conditions.

References

1. Wildiers H, Heeren P, et al. International Society of Geriatric Oncology consensus on geriatric assessment in older patients with cancer. J Clin Oncol. 2014;32:2595–603.
2. Liao X, Wang B, Kang Y. Novel coronavirus infection during the 2019-2020 epidemic: preparing intensive care units-the experience in Sichuan Province, China. Intensive Care Med. 2020;46(2):357–60. https://doi.org/10.1007/s00134-020-05954-2.
3. Meredith P, Inada-Kim M, Schmidt PE. A comparison of the quick sequential (sepsis-related) organ failure assessment score and the National Early Warning Score in non-ICU patients with/without infection. Crit Care Med. 2018;46(12):1923–33. https://doi.org/10.1097/CCM.0000000000003359.
4. Wu C, Chen X, Cai Y, Xia J, Zhou X, Xu S. Risk factors associated with acute respiratory distress syndrome and death in patients with coronavirus disease 2019 Pneumonia in Wuhan, China. JAMA Intern Med. 2020;180(7):934–43. https://doi.org/10.1001/jamainternmed.2020.0994.
5. Phua J, Weng L, Ling L, et al. Intensive care management of coronavirus disease 2019 (COVID-19): challenges and recommendations. Lancet Respir Med. 2020;8:P506–17. https://doi.org/10.1016/S2213-2600(20)30161-2.

The Management of Elderly Patients with COVID Out of the Hospital: The Italian Experience

22

Andrea Fabbo, Lucia Cavazzuti, Marilena De Guglielmo,
Paolo Giovanardi, Barbara Manni, Marina Turci,
Antonella Vaccina, and Andrea Spanò

22.1 Introduction

The coronavirus outbreak is drawing attention to older people as they are most exposed to infection and its dramatic consequences not only in the hospital but also in the community and nursing homes. Older people and especially the old-old, those with cognitive impairment and "frailty", especially elderly with various type of comorbidities, are the most vulnerable to the severe consequences of the disease [1]. Their clinical vulnerability is potentially exacerbated by the social phenomenon of ageism, where people are discriminated against solely based on their chronological age, and by discriminatory societal norms imposed by lockdown not always favourable to this population. Older people both at home and during hospitalisation or admission in long-term care facility suffer isolation and the lack of support of caregivers [2]. On 19th May, the AGE platform Europe releases the version of its report on COVID-19 and human rights concerns for older people. The description refers the situation regarding the respect of older people's human rights such as risks to the right to health, including mental health and palliative care, how digital exclusion adversely impacts older people's opportunities for social contact and access to

A. Fabbo (✉) · B. Manni · M. Turci · A. Vaccina
Geriatric Service, Cognitive Disorders and Dementia Unit, Health Authority and Services
(AUSL) of Modena, Modena, Italy
e-mail: a.fabbo@ausl.mo.it

L. Cavazzuti · M. De Guglielmo · P. Giovanardi
Specialised Outpatient Healthcare, Primary Care Department, Health Authority and Services
(AUSL) of Modena, Modena, Italy

A. Spanò
Medical Director of the Modena City District, Health Authority and Services (AUSL) of
Modena, Modena, Italy

195

N. Vargas, A. M. Esquinas (eds.), *Covid-19 Airway Management and Ventilation Strategy
for Critically Ill Older Patients*, https://doi.org/10.1007/978-3-030-55621-1_22

information, the increased risk of violence and abuse during the lockdown, the specific difficulties faced by older people in residential settings, those who live alone and those who receive care at home [3]. The burden of loneliness and social isolation can contribute to aggravating the clinical manifestations of COVID-19 disease and making it more difficult to manage especially in non-hospital settings where restrictions can be less implemented, known and accepted by health staff and family. The health emergency in which we find ourselves, which has affected at very different levels the Italian Regions, with a dramatic epicentre in those of the centre-north and more limited fallout in the South of the country [4], has highlighted that the main area for the management of patients with COVID-19 (especially the older patient) must be the national network. On the other hand, it has been evident for years, namely that territorial and home assistance has too often been neglected in favour of a more hospital-centric approach. In many Italian Regions, the primary care system and the instruments of the regional network are still too fragmented and without the coordination necessary to ensure effective continuity of hospital care in local context for the management of home patients. Just the emergency in progress has highlighted the need for a home care system no longer vertical silos with the different components managed as individual supplies of goods (technology) and services (hours of a nurse, device management) but with an integrated and transversal organisation based on taking care of patients, as many patient's and family associations had already requested. If in fact in some Regions are activated extraordinary measures for the home management of COVID patients, with innovative tools that until now were struggling to become systemic (think for example telemedicine and telemonitoring), these tools must be integrated into new organisational models aimed at the home management of chronic, multichronic and frail older patients. The experience and know-how of Homecare providers (which can be public or private in the context of a network of services) have become of fundamental importance for the home management of COVID patients (as well as all complex patients): from the home access of doctors and nurses to active surveillance, from telemonitoring with devices interconnected to the operations centre, from training to the use of PPE, up to the carrying out of swabs, samples and follow-up for patients discharged from hospitals [5, 6]. These activities require a strong presence on the territory and a previous organisational capacity, which make the Homecare providers a necessary actor for both general practitioners and hospital facilities to resign. Some Regions have promoted a specific measure for the management of patients at home such as USCA—Special Continuity of Care Unit established at the national level by a particular law due to COVID-19 emergency [7] or a specific model of home care as ADI–COVID (experienced in some Regions) which provides both home access of nursing workers and active surveillance remotely. Some providers of ADI (Integrated Home Care) have organised territorial teams of nurses dedicated exclusively to Adi COVID, to which it has freely chosen to support a medical centre of telemonitoring entirely composed of medical professionals, that daily receive and monitor (in close collaboration with the general practitioners to which they affect patients in the territory) the parameters of COVID patients in trust quarantine or recently discharged from hospitals.

22.2   Community Hospital

Community hospitals are intermediate structures between home care and hospital, essentially a bridge between national services and hospital for all those people who do not need to be hospitalised in acute wards or who need healthcare that they could not get at home. The persons admitted in this setting are especially older patients, mainly with chronic pathology, coming from a hospital, for acute or rehabilitative, that clinically can be discharged from hospitals for critical, but not in a condition to be adequately assisted at home. Community hospitals are therefore an essential instrument of hospital-territory integration and continuity of care, provided based on a comprehensive geriatric assessment (CGA) of the person to be assisted, through an integrated and individualised care plan. The assistance is provided in care modules, usually of 15–20 beds and the responsibility of the blade is a nursing manager. In contrast, the clinical responsibility is entrusted to family doctors or another doctor (for example, a specialist like a geriatrician). Nurses provide the assistance present continuously during the 24 h, assisted by other personnel (health and social workers) and other professionals (such as a therapist) when necessary. The average duration of the stay is limited, usually not to more than 6 weeks, about the evaluations and objectives defined [8]. In our experience at Castelfranco Emilia Community Hospital for only 2 months (two geriatricians and one cardiologist in integration work with a care team composed by nurses, physiotherapist and general practitioners) we managed 18 older patients (average age: 84 years); seven patients in the hospital became complicated by COVID infection for which not discharged, other three negatives were transferred waiting for discharge in clean settings. Upon discharge, 86% of patients returned home with a private assistant who was trained in mobilisation and health needs with video calls or in a room outside the ward. During the stay, there was a reduction in the severity of comorbidity with therapeutic adjustment and rehabilitation, a resolution of cases of delirium, an improvement in functional abilities (Barthel, Rankin) [9, 10] and reduction of the risk of pressure ulcers (Braden) [11]. We were able to remove the bladder catheter in half the cases. The drug therapy, because of therapeutic reconciliation, has been re-evaluated, for a reduction of behavioural disorders in cases of older adults with dementia. Atypical symptoms have been observed in our older patients with COVID-19.

Atypical symptoms of COVID-19 are described mainly in geriatrics and in patients with severe comorbidities (diabetes, hypertension, chronic obstructive pulmonary disease, cancer, dementia, degenerative disorders) [12]. Reports regarding COVID-19 atypical symptoms are growing even though many aspects of COVID-19 disease are unclear and a broad spectrum of not respiratory symptoms are described ranging from asymptomatic subjects to acute cardiovascular and not-cardiovascular diseases. The symptoms of COVID-19 are typical of respiratory nature such as fever, dry cough, flu, fatigue, and dyspnoea. The droplets are probably the most common way of transmission 1, and COVID-19 pneumonia has characteristic computed tomography abnormalities. A growing number of clinical evidence suggest that there might be other ways of transmission, such as the oral-faecal. Gastrointestinal symptoms such as nausea, vomiting, abdominal pain, discomfort, and diarrhoea have been observed, and a liver injury with a mild or moderate increase of amino-transferases has been frequently described. COVID-19 hepatotoxicity may be secondary to drug toxicity (antiviral medications, antibiotics, steroids). Still, the viral genome has been detected in salivary glands, in the gastrointestinal tract, and the liver tissue (hepatocytes and cholangiocytes) [13]. COVID-19 causes the overreaction of the immune system and has a great ability to activate the coagulation. These effects are responsible for acute disorders, increasing the chance of venous and arterial thrombotic events such as vein thrombosis, pulmonary embolisation, and arterial thrombosis [14, 15]. For example, Poissy and colleagues observed the appearance of pulmonary embolism in 20% of patient with severe CODID-19 infection admitted to the intensive care unit. In comparison, Stefanini and colleagues found the absence of coronary culprit lesions in 40% of COVID-19 patients with acute myocardial infarction 4.

Moreover, COVID-19 induces the synthesis of anticardiolipin antibodies and causes the damage to the vessel's wall, realising a vasculitis in small and in large vessels [16]. Also, a full spectrum of neurologic symptoms have been described in more than 35% of COVID-19 patients (dizziness, headache, impaired consciousness, ataxia, seizure, nerve pain, altered taste, smell, and vision), some of them with unclear pathogenesis, and not only due to cerebrovascular disease [17]. COVID-19 infection shows to be a multisystemic and complex disease. Evidence is growing, but many aspects are unclear, and a broad spectrum of not respiratory symptoms are described. Unusual symptoms may be present already from an early stage, and we do not know anything about the long-term impact of COVID-19 of many districts. In this epidemic period, great attention must be pointed to all unexplained symptoms, especially in geriatrics and in patients with comorbidities. Early diagnosis of COVID-19 would avoid the appearance of a cluster of cases, especially in patients with comorbidities.

22.3   Nursing Homes or Long-Term Care Facility

The WHO data on a global level, necessarily partial and under-sized because they collect only the cases confirmed by swab, estimate in over 80,000 deaths for COVID-19 in the elderly care homes in the world. At the press conference of 23 April 2020, the regional director of the World Health Organization for Europe Hans Kluge drew attention, according to European estimates, to the situation of the care homes, where deaths from the new coronavirus accounted for up to 50% in some countries. A «deeply worrying picture», added Kluge who tried to explain the reasons for such a tragedy: «the advanced age of patients, their basic health conditions, cognitive problems and hygiene advice due to intellectual disability or dementia, are all factors that put these people at greater risk. Also, many are prevented from receiving visits from family and friends and are sometimes subject to threats, abuse and abandonment. Equally worrying is how these care facilities operate, how patients receive care, which is providing pathways for the spread of the virus. It is important to remember that even very old and frail people, suffering from multiple chronic diseases, have a good chance of healing if they are well treated» [18]. The data of the ISS–Italian National Institute of Health (the only officially available on the subject, last updated to 14 April 2020) present a photograph at least critique. In the period 1 February–14 April deaths in Long-Term Care Facility or Nursing Home attributable to the virus were 40.2% of the total (2724 of the 6773 total deaths occurred in about 1000 structures, on the national panorama ISS counted 4629) with exception of some territories where it has reached higher peaks as PA Trento (78.8%), PA Bolzano (46.4%), Lombardy (53.4%) and Emilia-Romagna (57.7%) [19]. However, only 13.3% of the deaths related to coronavirus outbreak was determined by the swab. Looking at the currently active cases, if we consider only documented cases with a swab, we should have 1.43 cases per care homes with an incidence no higher than that of other social contexts; also including cases not confirmed by swab it comes to 4.3 cases per care homes. The problem of managing the older people with COVID-19 in the long-term care facility is a problem of great relevance all over the world; experts say nursing facilities are not well equipped to handle a pandemic such as COVID-19. The "coronavirus crisis" has revealed that little is still invested in these care settings both in terms of assistance and in terms of research in a sector that could make a great contribution to the knowledge of geriatric medicine [20]. We reported below some considerations based on our experience on the 52 Nursing Home (of which only 16 with COVID cases) of the province of Modena that we monitored and supported during the past 3 months. Isolation and quarantine are difficult to implement in these settings both because there is poor knowledge of the procedures to be adopted by the staff and because there is an objective difficulty in managing some types of older patients such as people living with dementia and behavioural disturbances; for example, people with COVID-19 positive who experience wandering are difficult to isolate, have difficulty wearing the protective mask and high risk of contaminating people and objects and need to be assisted in very large spaces with specially trained staff [21]. An observed risk was the possible drop-in care for non-COVID elderly as most staff were busy dealing with the emergency. In some cases care staff proved to be a scarce resource during this period, both because it was impossible to train him or pass on the missing skills in such a short time (especially on health procedures), and because absenteeism phenomena have arisen in some contexts for fear of operators or movements of personnel between Nursing Homes and Public Health linked to extraordinary hires from Regions occurring in parallel. An important issue to consider is the relationship with family members. They are often afraid that some truths (especially about the virus) may be hidden from them, so they need reassurance and transparency about the health of their loved ones. Another aspect to consider was the relationship between Nursing Home and hospital; often, this relationship, where the structure is not part of a social-health service network, is problematic. During the epidemic, given the scarcity of hospital beds, the need to stratify these patients was also strengthened to guarantee the most appropriate treatments. For this reason, it is essential to introduce validated tools for the prognosis in the Nursing home care practice: they are necessary for hospitalisation, the optimisation of pharmacological and non-pharmacological therapies, rehabilitation and palliative care. First of all, they are also important from a medico-legal point of view. In Chap. 14 we have already discussed with the issue of using tools necessary to guarantee comprehensive geriatric assessment (CGA) also and above all for prognostic purposes such as the Multi Prognostic Index—MPI [22, 23] or the Clinical Frailty Scale [24]. Palliative care is another crucial issue in Long-term Care Facility. In recent years there has been a slow introduction of palliative care in these care settings; in most cases, palliative care that aims at the quality of life instead of prolonging life is well accepted in the nursing care homes also because it is often supported by the care staff (doctors, nurses, psychologists, educators) and in some cases meet the wishes and needs of the older people who live inside [25]. For these reasons, we have formalised a care pathway for older people with COVID-19 in-home care facilities (LCF) with aims of (a) managing COVID-19 positive older patient in LCF with available treatments and monitoring the evolution of the disease also with the use of telemedicine tools; (b) reducing improper access to the hospital to dedicate intensive settings to patients with the most appropriate indications; (c) humanise the inevitable death of very frail older adults with COVID pneumonia 19 facilitating the delivery of palliative care. The strategies adopted were of two types: first to network all the nursing care homes with the Health Authority and Services of Modena and after to develop a series of accompanying actions such as directing and supporting the treatment actions of nursing home staff by support healthcare professionals: geriatricians, palliatives, infectious disease specialists and psychologists (especially for the part relating to sharing, communication and support of the family members). The protocol provided indications and tools for the care team and communication methods for family members in according to the WHO guidance Integrated care for older people (ICOPE) for the person-centred and coordinated model of care [26] and the WHO guide Integrating palliative care and symptom relief into responses to humanitarian emergencies and crises [27, 28]. Palliative care including relief of symptoms and social support should be practised by all the healthcare staff and social workers in the nursing home for older persons affected by COVID-19 just as it is important to invite older persons to discuss advance care plans to determine their priorities and preferences [29]. Indications for care staff provided by our clinical pathway were: to prepare a classification of the older patients based on biological and clinical frailty and a possible indication for palliative care based on Clinical Frailty Scale (CFS) [24] according to NICE guidelines [30], to communicate in advance to the family members the condition of the frailty of the older patient and the absence of indication for hospitalisation in case of pneumonia from COVID-19 as well as the possibility of inclusion in a palliative/end-of-life path, to provide indications for both curative and palliative treatment in Nursing Home facility, and to help in the diagnosis of COVID-19 even in the presence of atypical symptoms. At the same time, it was important to provide tools to Nursing Home such as personal protective equipment

(PPE) for healthcare staff engaged in assistance in COVID environments, availability of oxygen-therapy by facilitating and speeding up the supply routes, availability of necessary drugs (Chloroquine but also Morphine and Benzodiazepines with related continuous infusion products), geriatric consultants for the management of delirium (with pharmacological and non-pharmacological methods), expert consultants in Palliative Care through proactive and structured telephone contacts or, where necessary, with team supervision in a "clean" environment), a practical vademecum for the treatment of the main symptoms and a telemedicine monitoring project of parameters for the emergency management of COVID-19 with a direct connection to the Emergency Room to decide on possible hospitalisation if necessary. Regarding the pharmacological treatment of older patient with COVID-19 in Nursing home care facility, we followed the existing published literature, which, for the most part is observational, with few clinical trials. For example, the treatment with hydroxychloroquine (widely used in non-hospital settings, with or without azithromycin association) is an empirical therapy of COVID-19, and it has a limited duration (5–7 days) [31–33]. Considering the preliminary and limited evidence to date, the empirical treatment with hydroxychloroquine for the treatment of COVID-19 must provide a careful evaluation of the risks/benefits and chronic pathologies (long QT syndrome, heart failure, ischemic heart disease, insufficiency kidney or liver, electrolyte disturbances) and potentially adverse events, especially in older and frail patients. In Nursing home to monitor patients at high risk of QT interval elongation, we consider serial control of ECG and electrolyte mostly in older patients with diuretic and renal failure therapy. In the early stages of the epidemic, off-label use of hydroxychloroquine was allowed, based on the data preliminaries available, only in the context of the national emergency management plan COVID-19; in light of the evidence from literature recently produced, AIFA (Italian Regulatory Agency for drugs) has suspended authorisation for off-label use of the drug outside of clinical trials [34, 35]. In our protocol we consider very important for an older patient with COVID-19 in Nursing Home the support treatment based on hydration to maintain an adequate, effective circulating volume, prophylaxis with LMWH (low-molecular-weight heparin) especially for elderly with limited motor activity, need for antibiotic therapy if signs and symptoms of a bacterial infection occur (for example, urinary tract infections in patients with bladder catheters, clinical deterioration of a previous respiratory picture attributed to COVID-19 by respiratory superinfection with possible bacterial aetiology), and administration of vitamin D supplementation already planned for institutionalised people to counter the deficiency. It is also essential a review of medication prescriptions to reduce in older patient polypharmacy and prevent drugs interactions and adverse events to those being treated with COVID-19 disease [36].

A practical scheme of possible pharmacological treatments is indicated in Table 22.1.

Table 22.1 COVID-19 therapy for older patients in nursing home[a]

Drug	Use	Contraindications
Hydroxychloroquine	Likely efficacy in mild forms; controversial use	QTc prolongation, drugs interactions, dysphagia
Macrolides	For bacterial superinfections	Many and multiple adverse events, drugs interactions
Corticosteroids	Poor studies, not recommended	Many adverse events
LMWH	In therapeutic doses	Bleeding, difficulty of checks
Hydration	High risk of dehydration in COVID-19 older patients	Heart failure
Oxygen-therapy	Dyspnoea	Low flows are not effective, aerosols

[a]Adapted from Nicola Veronese, geriatrician, Webinar SIGOT (Italian Geriatric Society of Hospital and Territory): The elderly and COVID-19 pandemic: epidemiology and clinic in different care settings, on May 17th, 2020

22.4 The Management of Older People with COVID-19 in Dementia Special Care Unit

Dementia is a syndrome consisting of several symptoms that include a reduced ability to perform familiar tasks, impairment of memory, judgement and reasoning and changes in mood and behaviour. Persons with dementia are still able to sense, feel and appreciate lived spaces, and they are less distressed if the lived spaces are familiar and comfortable. Moreover, persons living with dementia experience a reduction in their lived space as dementia develops [37]. The feeling of unfamiliarity increases with the symptoms of dementia. There is considerable evidence that a person-centred approach can improve quality of life for these persons. A person-centred approach is about connecting with others, building and maintaining relationships, embracing uniqueness and the expression of this, and providing a safe, supportive environment with high levels of dignity and respect for those within the environment. Older people with dementia need to live in situations that preserve four important needs: belonging, meaningfulness safety and security and autonomy. Sustain person-centred care means to support the physical, social and environmental dimensions. There is ample evidence the services and supports designed and delivered in a way that is integrated collaborative and mutually respectful of all persons improve quality of life and reduce disability and the appearance of behavioural disorders [38]. In this view, people with dementia are active participants in their care and family members play an important role in ensuring well-being of their relative. There are different types of care facilities for elderly subjects suffering from dementia. There is a general view that special care units with trained personnel are the most appropriate environment to enhance the quality of care for subjects who suffer from dementia and carry on the person-centred model. They are specially designed for patients with dementia, implying resident security and safety through locking systems, signposts and communal living areas. The staff is specially trained to deal with behavioural and psychological symptoms of dementia. This specialisation results in better-organised care offered by special units, compared to traditional nursing homes and in more family involvement. Usually, these special units do not accept a large number of patients to offer a more home-like experience to residents. Care providers in these units follow a vision of long-term care by emphasising normalisation of daily life [39]. At the beginning of 2020, a new outbreak was reported, and quickly the infection spread for the whole world. Infections are a leading cause of morbidity and mortality among nursing home residents. Therefore, identifying effective practices to reduce infection transmission is necessary to manage health outcomes and costs [40]. Older adults are very vulnerable at the onset of coronavirus disease pandemic. How to manage people with dementia during this pandemic situation has raised great concerns [41]. In a nursing home, if there is a person infected, isolation precautions are recommended to prevent the spread of pathogens between other residents and staff. This practice includes confining an infected resident to a private room and let him or her there for all the period he/she is contagious. Furthermore, he sleeps, eats, spends all days and nights in his bedroom with restricted social contacts. Further isolation has well-established negative psychological effects. Particularly in a person with dementia can increase confusion and behavioural disorders and facilitate the appearance of delirium that is a risk condition also for the typical hypoxia and the use of some medications to contrast COVID infection. Quarantine and isolation are highly effective tools in the control of infections, but they have been difficult to implement effectively in nursing homes, especially in setting as Dementia Care Unit [42]. In particular, the perception the infection control practices seem in conflict with quality of life goals and rights of the residents. People living with dementia might have difficulties in remembering safeguard procedures, such as wearing masks, washing hands or avoid personal contacts, so it is more difficult to protect themselves. Their compromised cognitive functioning, insight and judgement impact their capacity to comply with restrictions. Moreover, complementary treatments or non-pharmacological therapies such as occupational activities, multisensory stimulation like massage and face-to-face communication must be reduced or abolished. Autonomy reduction, less meaningful activities and less social contacts lead towards an increase of confusion and challenging behaviour and reduce the independence of the patient. It is also important to remember that some drugs used to treat the SARS Cov 2 pneumonia are associated with neuropsychiatric adverse effects. They can also have life-threatening interactions with psychotropic drugs leading to increased toxicity and undesirable side-effects, such as QT interval prolongation. Guidelines for the infection prevention and control in nursing homes, written before COVID emergency, considered acceptable the possibility to cohorting (create a group of residents with the same infection during all activities to prevent organisms transmission to unaffected patients) [43]. This action could be a good compromise to benefits and drawbacks of isolation to establish best practices. The same difficulty arises in psychiatric contests, and different situation hospitals created separated wards for COVID positive patients with psychiatric illnesses [44, 45]. If there are some COVID-19 cases in particularly in special unit care for demented people, as documented by our experience at the Dementia Unit of the Nursing Home "il Carpine" of the city of Carpi, could be very useful to share the accessible space in a COVID-in and COVID-free areas where people can move free minimising risks and preserving freedom and independence. On the base of this strategy, widespread screening may be required to have the new possibility to identify all positive residents, symptomatic and asymptomatic who need to be isolated [46, 47]. Within the COVID area with people with dementia, the challenge is to manage the infections risks and maintain personal dignity. This prerogative is difficult but possible, and it is important to observe more rules. First of all, should be avoid all visits in the area from relatives or friends and nonessential personnel. Staff should be provided with facial masks and all necessary equipment to assist properly and minimise risks. The staff must receive all information about the infection and the control practices and understand the importance of variations in daily practice. On the other hand, the staff should not forget the main principles of best care practice for people with dementia and find a compromise between the two and create new solutions. The level of anxiety among staff in nursing homes is high, and they develop signs of exhaustion after a prolonged time at work wearing uncomfortable protected tools and observing suffering residents. Managing people with dementia and behavioural disorders create a major logistical challenge. Education, some breaks and psychological support could be important tools to prevent the burnout. The psychologist can provide online consultation for the staff and patients' relatives. During the day, older patients who are asymptomatic or have few symptoms could go out from their bedrooms and move in a dining room or, if accessible and the clinical conditions permit, in a garden. The environment should be essential than usual, with less furniture and stuff, easy to clean. It is not necessary to avoid completely used non-pharmacological activities, but it is possible to choose those activities without direct physical interactions such as listen to music, watch movies, read newspapers or novels. It is also important to maintain physical distance as much as possible. Occupational activities could also be provided. A strategy to avoid manipulation of materials from a resident to another could be the creation of personal boxes for every resident. These boxes could be filled with favourited materials that will be used only to one person such as clothes, colouring pages and pencils, newspapers and so on. The organisation of space creating a separated facility for COVID-positive patients permits the possibility to move freely in the COVID area; to have different night and day spaces and go on with meaningful activities this organisation helps demented residents not to develop delirium, sleep disorders, challenging behaviours and hypomobility syndrome. Moreover the staff is less anxious, preserves a better relationship with the residents, and it is more satisfying. Communication should be maintained with all residents. If a patient has got hearing impairment, worsened from the use of masks, could be introduced the use of blackboards or paper to write on. Physical restraint and pharmacological sedation measures should be the last tool to use in a person-centred view. Family members have an important role in person-centred care with people with dementia. Staff must create a partnership with the patient relatives to share his/her individualised assistance plan and explain how the assistance to all the COVID area will be provided. Families are beset by fear and anxiety as COVID-19 makes inroads at nursing homes across the country, threatening the lives of vulnerable older adults. It is important to permit to stay in touch with loved ones via telephone calls or video visits. If the COVID area is at the ground floor could be possible organise visits from the window. Scheduling a time for a call, a video chat or a "window visit" may make it easier. Frequent contacts with the staff can also be useful as well as a phone call with the psychologist.

22.5   The Management at Home: The Role of USCA (Special Care Unit of Continuity of Care)

According to the guidelines published by the World Health Organization [48] the decision to monitor patients with mild COVID-19 in a community facility or home it should be assessed on a case-by-case based on local care pathways or the existing service network. The decision may depend on the severity of the disease, the request for supportive care, the risk of complications and the conditions of care at home, including the presence of vulnerable persons in the family context [49]. USCA (Special Care Unit of Continuity of care) are teams formed by general practitioners, specialists and nurses, with a specific task: to identify and assist, at home, people with COVID-19. They do not need to be hospitalised. Only in Emilia Romagna Region n° 77 USCA are active, involving over 400 doctors and 85 nurses. In total, there are more than 20,000 benefits provided: not only tampons but also, for example, electrocardiograms, pulmonary ultrasounds, administration of therapies and visits to older people in nursing homes. In Modena compared to other regional provinces, the USCA's team have operated less in a nursing home due to the presence of the support team (geriatricians, infectious disease specialists and palliatives) foreseen in our path of taking care of an older patient with COVID previously described (for example in Modena we have only n° 149 interventions of USCA in Nursing Home versus n° 2.618 interventions of Reggio Emilia or n°1093 responses of Piacenza) [50]. In this way, it was possible to intercept the disease, support family doctors in the home care of their patients with coronavirus and relieve the pressure on the hospital network. The main aim of the USCA is to assist at-home patients with COVID-19 who do not need hospitalisation; in this way, hospitals are lightened, while general practitioners can continue to follow ordinary patients. Specialists can take part, those who are still taking the course to become a doctor of General Medicine and newly qualified waiting to take part in the competition to enter a specialisation school. Why are young people privileged? It is not only a matter of lack of workforce but also a way to protect older doctors who are more exposed to the risks that a SARS-Cov-2 infection can entail. The USCA team is activated by the general practitioner while the person cannot call them directly. They are active from Monday to Sunday and from 8:00 am to 8.00 pm, although there may be time variations depending on the zones of Italy. Their purpose is not to make swabs, but to intervene when an already positive patient, or strongly suspected of having contracted the COVID-19 needs medical assistance. Specifically, the USCA team will come when:

(a) A positive person has mild symptoms (such as cough and fever at 37.5°), but is over 70 years old or already suffers from previous diseases
(b) One person was hospitalised, but then discharged from hospital with a diagnosis of COVID-19, to await a recovery in home isolation
(c) A person has a high fever that has been going on for at least 4 days or has difficulty breathing, even if it is not officially positive.

Once the family doctor has made a telephone triage, the unit is sent to the patient's home, naturally equipped with all personal protective equipment (PPE) that must be provided directly from the Health Authority. At this point, he visits the patient, recording all the parameters and above all measuring his saturation with an oximeter: a fundamental value to understand whether or not hospitalisation is necessary. The USCA team also perform a pulmonary ultrasound; this is especially important for suspected cases because if pneumonia is in its early stages, the X-ray could even be harmful, while the ultrasound can reveal if there is lung damage giving a big help to decide whether the patient should be treated at home or sent to the hospital. In the period included from April 20th to May 25th 2020, the USCA of Modena (n° 3.678 cases of COVID-19 as of May 1, equal to 0.52 per cent of the population) followed n° 1939 patients (medium age 63 years; range 55–88 years) through various types of activities: telephone triage (n° 870), home care visits (n° 697), visits in Nursing Home (n° 203) pharmacological interventions (n° 122) and other activities (n° 60) as swabs, electrocardiogram, and pulmonary ultrasound.

22.6　Conclusive Remarks

The experience conducted in the network of services has shown us that it is possible to manage the elderly with COVID in settings other than the hospital, but this is only achieved when the health services (from acute care hospital to the system of intermediate care to Nursing homes and home care services) are interconnected, and attention is not fragmented. The separation of the flows of COVID and non-COVID patients must permeate the entire care process not only inside but also outside the hospital. Many public Health Agencies (like ours in Modena) have defined COVID patient discharge paths in structures dedicated to lower levels of intensity of care (small care), COVID patient hotel (i.e., hospitalisation places) dedicated to stable but still positive COVID patients. The latter cannot be discharged directly at home in order not to create further conditions of contagion. Also, the presence of a network of services coordinated by the Health Authority has made it possible to manage the older patients in various care settings such as the community hospital, the Nursing homes (including services dedicated to people living with dementia) and the home care through the experience of the USCA. The emergency highlighted the high potential of the technology and a relative speed of adoption both for the needs of COVID patients (tools for assistance and monitoring, tele-diagnostics, etc.), and to guarantee safety to patients who need care or health control activities (e.g., telemedicine and teleconsultation). The diffusion of these technologies in the health system is still scarce. It is necessary to strengthen these tools to make them available not only in times of crisis but to integrate them as ordinary tools to support the delivery of health services also in the following stages of the pandemic.

References

1. Lauretani F, Ravazzoni G, Roberti MF, Longobucco Y, Adorni E, Grossi M, De Iorio A, La Porta U, Fazio C, Gallini E, Federici R, Salvi M, Ciarrocchi E, Rossi F, Bergamin M, Bussolati G, Grieco I, Broccoli F, Zucchini I, Ielo G, Morganti S, Artoni A, Arisi A, Tagliaferri S, Maggio M. Assessment and treatment of older individuals with COVID 19 multi-system

disease: clinical and ethical implications. Acta Bio Med. 2020;91(2). Available from https://www.mattioli1885journals.com/index.php/actabiomedica/article/view/9629.

2. Simard J, Volicer L. Loneliness and isolation in long-term care and the Covid-19 pandemic. J Am Med Dir Assoc. 2020; https://doi.org/10.1016/j.jamda.2020.05.006.

3. https://www.age-platform.eu/publications/covid-19-and-human-rights-concerns-older-persons.

4. Istituto Superiore di Sanità Epidemia COVID-19 Aggiornamento nazionale 26 maggio 2020. https://www.epicentro.iss.it/coronavirus/bollettino/Bollettino-sorveglianza-integrata-COVID-19_26-maggio-2020.pdf.

5. Baxter S, Johnson M, Chambers D, Sutton A, Goyder E, Booth A. Understanding new models of integrated care in developed countries: a systematic review. Southampton, UK: NIHR Journals Library; 2018.

6. Zonneveld N, Driessen N, Stüssgen RAJ, Minkman MMN. Values of integrated care: a systematic review. Int J Integr Care. 2018;18(4):9. https://doi.org/10.5334/ijic.4172.

7. D. L. 9 marzo 2020, n. 14 Disposizioni urgenti per il potenziamento del Servizio sanitario nazionale in relazione all'emergenza COVID-19, art 8. Istituzione, per la durata dello stato di emergenza di Unità Speciali di Continuità Assistenziale (di seguito anche USCA) per la gestione domiciliare dei pazienti affetti da COVID-19 che non necessitano di ricovero ospedaliero.

8. Fantini MP, Pieri G, Rosa S, Caruso B, Rossi A, Pianori D, Longo F. Definire e programmare le Cure Intermedie nella filiera dei servizi per la fragilità e gli anziani: metodi ed evidenze dal caso della Regione Emilia-Romagna. Mecosan Manag Econom Sanitaria. 2015;93:75–97.

9. Sainsbury A, Seebass G, Bansal A, Young JB. Reliability of the Barthel index when used with older people. Age Ageing. 2005;34(3):228–32. https://doi.org/10.1093/ageing/afi063.

10. Bruno A, Shah N, Lin C, et al. Improving modified Rankin scale assessment with a simplified questionnaire. Stroke. 2010;41(5):1048–50. https://doi.org/10.1161/STROKEAHA.109.571562.

11. Stotts NA, Gunningberg L. How to try this: predicting pressure ulcer risk. Am J Nurs. 2007;107(11):40–8. http://www.nursingcenter.con/lnc/cearticle?tid=751548. Accessed 19 May 2014.

12. Zhu N, Zhang D, Wang W, et al. A novel coronavirus from patients with pneumonia in China. N Engl J Med. 2020;382:727–33. https://doi.org/10.1056/NEJMoa2001017.

13. Gu J, Han B, Wang J. COVID-19: gastrointestinal manifestations and potential fecal-oral transmission. Gastroenterology. 2020;158(6):1518–9. https://doi.org/10.1053/j.gastro.2020.02.054.

14. Xie Y, Wang X, Yang P, Zhang S. COVID-19 complicated by acute pulmonary embolism. Radiol Cardiothor Imag. 2020;2:e200067. https://doi.org/10.1148/ryct.2020200067.

15. Zhang Y, Xiao M, Zhang S, et al. Coagulopathy and antiphospholipid antibodies in patients with Covid-19. N Engl J Med. 2020;382:e38. https://doi.org/10.1056/NEJMc2007575.

16. Poissy J, Goulay J, Captan M, et al. Pulmonary embolism in COVID-19 patients: awareness of an increased prevalence. Circulation. 2020; https://doi.org/10.1161/CIRCULATIONAHA.120.047430.

17. Mao L, Jin H, Wang M, Hu Y, et al. Neurologic manifestations of hospitalized patients with coronavirus disease 2019 in Wuhan, China. JAMA Neurol. 2020;77(6):683–90. https://doi.org/10.1001/jamaneurol.2020.1127.

18. Chidambaram P. Kaiser Family Foundation Issue Brief: state reporting of cases and deaths due to COVID-19 in long-term care facilities. https://www.kff.org/medicaid/issuebrief/state-reporting-of-cases-and-deaths-due-tocovid-19-in-long-term-care-facilities/. Accessed 26 April 2020.

19. https://www.epicentro.iss.it/coronavirus/sars-cov-2-survey-rsa.

20. Grabowski DC, Mor V. Nursing home care in crisis in the wake of COVID-19. JAMA. 2020;324:23–4. https://doi.org/10.1001/jama.2020.8524.

21. https://www.scie.org.uk/care-providers/coronavirus-covid-19/dementia/care-homes.

22. Pilotto A, Cella A, Pilotto A, et al. Three decades of comprehensive geriatric assessment evidence coming from different healthcare settings and specific clinical conditions. J Am Med Dir Assoc. 2017;18(2):192.e1–e11.

23. Zucchelli A, Vetrano DL, Grande G, et al. Comparing the prognostic value of geriatric health indicators: a population-based study. BMC Med. 2019;17:185. https://doi.org/10.1186/s12916-019-1418-2.

24. Rockwood K, Song X, MacKnight C, et al. A global clinical measure of fitness and frailty in elderly people. CMAJ. 2005;173(5):489–95. https://doi.org/10.1503/cmaj.050051.

25. Hall S, Kolliakou A, Petkova H, Froggatt K, Higginson IJ. Interventions for improving palliative care for older people living in nursing care homes. Cochrane Database Syst Rev. 2011;2011(3):CD007132. https://doi.org/10.1002/14651858.CD007132.pub2.

26. World Health Organization. Integrated care for older people (ICOPE): Guidelines on community-level interventions to manage declines in intrinsic capacity. Geneva: World Health Organization; 2017. https://apps.who.int/iris/bitstream/handle/10665/258981/9789241550109-eng.pdf;j

27. World Health Organization. Guide Integrating palliative care and symptom relief into responses to humanitarian emergencies and crises. Geneva: World Health Organization; 2018. https://www.who.int/publications-detail/integrating-palliative-care-and-symptom-relief-into-the-response-to-humanitarian-emergencies-and-crises.

28. Krakauer EL, Daubman BR, Aloudat T, Bhadelia N, Black L, Janjanin S, et al. Palliative care needs of people affected by natural hazards, political or ethnic conflict, epidemics of life-threatening infections, and other humanitarian crises. In: Waldman E, Glass M, editors. A field manual for palliative care in humanitarian crises. New York: Oxford; 2020. p. 4–13.

29. Di Luca A, et al. Law on advance health care directives: a medical perspective. La Clinica Terapeutica. 2018;169(2):e77–81. ISSN 1972-6007. Available at https://www.clinicaterapeutica.it/ojs/index.php/ClinicaTerapeutica/article/view/150.

30. COVID-19 rapid guideline: critical care in adults NICE guideline. Published: 20 March 2020. www.nice.org.uk/guidance/ng159.

31. Chen J, Lui D, Liu L, Lui P, Xu Q, Xia L, et al. A pilot study of hydroxychloroquine in treatment of patients with moderate COVID-19. J Zhejiang Univ (Med Sci). 2020;49(2):215–9. https://doi.org/10.3785/j.issn.1008-9292.2020.03.03.

32. Gautret P, Lagier JC, Parola P, Hoang VT, Meddeb L, Mailhe M, et al. Hydroxychloroquine and azithromycin as a treatment of COVID-19: results of an open-label non-randomized clinical trial. Int J Antimicrob Agents. 2020;2020:105949.

33. Gautret P, Lagier JC, Parola P, Hoang VT, Meddeb L, Sevestre J, et al. Clinical and microbiological effect of a combination of hydroxychloroquine and azithromycin in 80 COVID-19 patients with at least a six-day follow up: a pilot observational study. Travel Med Infect Dis. 2020;2020:101663.

34. Mehra MR, Desai SS, Ruschitzka F, Patel AN. Hydroxychloroquine or chloroquine with or without a macrolide for treatment of COVID-19: a multinational registry analysis. Lancet. 2020; https://doi.org/10.1016/S0140-6736(20)31180-6. https://www.thelancet.com/journals/lancet/article/PIIS0140-6736(20)31180-6/fulltext.

35. https://www.aifa.gov.it/documents/20142/1123276/idrossiclorochina_29.05.2020.pdf/3958aea0-5a5f-2d05-b1f6-034dbe28ce2a.

36. Nagham A, Sarah H, Lisa K, Rhiannon B, Emily R. COVID-19 pandemic: considerations for safe medication use in older adults with multimorbidity and polypharmacy. J Gerontol Ser A Biol Sci Med Sci. 2020; https://doi.org/10.1093/gerona/glaa104.

37. Førsund LH, Grov EK, Helvik A-S, Juvet LK, Skovdahl K, Eriksen S. The experience of lived space in persons with dementia: a systematic meta-synthesis. BMC Geriatr. 2018;18:33.

38. Ballard C, Corbett A, Orrell M, Williams G, Moniz-Cook E, Romeo R, Woods B, Garrod L, Testad I, Woodward-Carlton B, Wenborn J, Knapp M, Fossey J. Ballard C, et al impact of person-centred care training and person-centred activities on quality of life, agitation, and anti-psychotic use in people with dementia living in nursing homes: a cluster-randomised controlled trial. PLoS Med. 2018 Feb 6;15(2):e1002500. https://doi.org/10.1371/journal.pmed.1002500.

39. Kok JS, Berg IJ, Scherder EJ. Special care units and traditional care in dementia: relationship with behavior, cognition, functional status and quality of life—a review. Dement Geriatr Cogn Dis Extra. 2013;3(1):360–75. https://doi.org/10.1159/000353441.

40. Cohen CC, Pogorzelska-Maziarz M, Herzig CT, et al. Infection prevention and control in nursing homes: a qualitative study of decision-making regarding isolation-based practices. BMJ Qual Saf. 2015;24(10):630–6. https://doi.org/10.1136/bmjqs-2015-003952.
41. Wang H, Li T, Barbarino P, Gauthier S, Brodaty H, Molinuevo JL, Xie H, Sun Y, Yu E, Tang Y, Weidner W, Yu X. Dementia care during COVID-19. Lancet. 2020;395(10231):1190–1. https://doi.org/10.1016/S0140-6736(20)30755-8.
42. Iaboni A, Cockburn A, Marcil M, Rodrigues K, Marshall C, Garcia MA, Quirt H, Reynolds KB, Keren R, Flint AJ. Achieving safe, effective and compassionate quarantine or isolation of older adults with dementia in nursing homes. Am J Geriatr Psychiatry. 2020; https://doi.org/10.1016/j.jagp.2020.04.025.
43. World Health Organization. Prevention and control of outbreaks of seasonal influenza in long-term care facilities: a review of the evidence and best-practice guidance. 2017. http://www.euro.who.int/__data/assets/pdf_file/0015/330225/LTCF-best-practice.
44. Xiang YT, Zhao YJ, Liu ZH, Li XH, Zhao N, Cheung T, Ng CH. The COVID-19 outbreak and psychiatric hospitals in China: managing challenges through mental health service reform. Int J Biol Sci. 2020;16(10):1741–4. https://doi.org/10.7150/ijbs.45072.
45. Hernández-Huerta D, Alonso-Sánchez EB, Carrajo-Garcia CA, Montes-Rodríguez JM. The impact of COVID-19 on acute psychiatric inpatient unit. Psychiatry Res. 2020;290:113107. https://doi.org/10.1016/j.psychres.2020.113107.
46. Arons MM, Hatfield KM, Reddy SC, Kimball A, James A, Jacobs JR, Taylor J, Spicer K, Bardossy AC, Oakley LP, Tanwar S, Dyal JW, Harney J, Chisty Z, Bell JM, Methner M, Paul P, Carlson CM, McLaughlin HP, Thornburg N, Tong S, Tamin A, Tao Y, Uehara A, Harcourt J, Clark S, Brostrom-Smith C, Page LC, Kay M, Lewis J, Montgomery P, Stone ND, Clark TA, Honein MA, Duchin JS, Jernigan JA, for the Public Health–Seattle and King County and CDC COVID-19 Investigation Team*. Presymptomatic SARS-CoV-2 Infections and Transmission in a Skilled Nursing Facility. N Engl J Med. 2020;382(22):2081–90. https://doi.org/10.1056/NEJMoa2008457.
47. Brown EE, Kumar S, Rajji TK, Pollock BG, Mulsant BH. Anticipating and mitigating the impact of the COVID-19 pandemic on Alzheimer's disease and related dementias. Am J Geriatr Psychiatry. 2020;28(7):712–21. https://doi.org/10.1016/j.jagp.2020.04.010.
48. Clinical Management of Covid-19, Interim guidance, Geneva: World Health Organization, 2020 WHO reference number: WHO/2019-nCoV/clinical/2020.5. https://apps.who.int/iris/bitstream/handle/10665/332196/WHO-2019-nCoV-clinical-2020.5-eng.pdf?sequence=1&isAllowed=y. Accessed 27 May 2020.
49. Home care for patients with COVID-19 presenting with mild symptoms and management of their contacts. Geneva: World Health Organization, 2020. https://www.who.int/publications-detail/home-care-for-patients-with-suspected-novel-coronavirus-(ncov)-infection-presenting-with-mild-symptoms-and-management-of-contacts.
50. Regione Emilia-Romagna: report attività delle USCA. https://salute.regione.emilia-romagna.it/notizie/regione/2020/maggio/cure-al-domicilio-per-i-pazienti-covid-19-in-emilia-romagna-sono-attive-81-unita-speciali-di-continuita-assistenziale-usca.

Part VI

Conclusion

The Geriatric Perspectives in the Time of COVID-19

23

Nicola Vargas, Loredana Tibullo, and Antonio M. Esquinas

23.1 Introduction

During the COVID-19 pandemic, the considerable preponderance of deaths is occurring in older persons. The current Italian data, for example, indicate that persons aged 70 years and older contribute to about 85% of the death events [1]. In the scenario of rationing the resources, the differentiation between the causes of death can be difficult. Specifically, to establish if the death of an older patient is due to COVID-19 or the result of treatment limitations can be difficult [2]. The reading of actual pandemic from the geriatric point of view should include different planes: ethical, legal and clinical.

23.2 Ethical Factors

The caring decision-making process is becoming more difficult during an epidemic. The first reason is that the choice of who have to care it has fallen mainly on the physician's shoulders. They found with few intensive care beds but with many admissions of severe patients with acute respiratory failure. The ventilators were lacking too. Physicians excluded then from ICU older patients as the great emergency requires and as some scientific societies such as SIAARTI have suggested in the recommendations of 2020 [3]. Many commentators in many

N. Vargas (✉)
Geriatric and Intensive Geriatric Cares, San Giuseppe Moscati Hospital, Avellino, Italy

L. Tibullo
Medicine Department, Ward of Internal Medicine, San Giuseppe Moscati Hospital, Aversa, Italy

A. M. Esquinas
Intensive Care Unit, Hospital Morales Meseguer, Murcia, Spain

N. Vargas, A. M. Esquinas (eds.), *Covid-19 Airway Management and Ventilation Strategy for Critically Ill Older Patients*, https://doi.org/10.1007/978-3-030-55621-1_23

newspapers have considered these recommendations ethically wrong. From geriatrics, society can give more value to persons, independently of their age [4]. Many elders are fit or very fit. In seven and eight decades, many older adults occupy essential positions in society. The risk that these people are excluded only for their age and life expectancy evaluation is very high. But if we make age the unique criterion for rationing, we take a giant step towards overt valuing of some lives over others [5].

23.3   Legal Aspects

Informed consent for clinical treatment is a vital part of contemporary medical practice. In everyday clinical practice, physicians are required by law to obtain informed consent and dissent in many different clinical situations, including individualised elderly care planning, rehabilitation planning, means of protection, surgical procedures, diagnostic tests and other invasive procedures and techniques [6]. A community who can save young and the elderly is also a community that respects the legal right to have the possibility of choice, when competent, or to give the chance of choice to the family members or legally surrogate. In Europe, in England for example, there is the possibility that healthcare practitioners may give therapy without the consent of a patient or their legal representative. The justification for doing this is that the procedure is "necessary". However, the concept of "necessity" does not only apply in emergencies but can justify routine treatment and even simple care, although delivering treatment deemed necessary by the medical profession [7]. During pandemic in the case of the allocation of scarce therapeutic interventions and resources, Persad et al. in 2009 [8] proposed the "complete lives system" that incorporates five principles: youngest-first, prognosis, save the most lives, lottery and instrumental value. As such, it prioritises younger people who have not yet lived a complete life and will be unlikely to do so without aid. The complete lives system also considers prognosis since it aims to achieve full lives. A young person with a poor prognosis has had few life-years but lacks the potential to live a complete life. Considering prognosis forestalls the concern that disproportionately large amounts of resources will be directed to young people with poor prognoses. Rather than saving the most lives, prognosis allocation aims to keep the most life-years. But are the most life-years a reasonable value? A person with his life has legal rights. The system proposed intended to avoid futility medicine and waste resources in case of an expected negative outcome.

23.4   The Clinical Context

During the COVID-19 pandemic, the necessity of multidisciplinary evaluation of the patients remains the main road. In this way, physicians, family members, psychologists and palliative physicians could establish an agreed advance individualised plan. Until now, all of these perspectives have failed. Family members have been excluded from the decision-making process from the limitations of the pandemic. The less time available and the overworking of physicians do not allow the possibility to make a multidisciplinary evaluation. The SIAARTI recommendations intended to help physicians in these emergencies. SIAARTI decision doesn't disturb us. From a clinical point of view, beyond ethical and social issues, the problem starts from afar. Every day in clinical practice, for many years, before the actual pandemic, we come across older patients with clinical or a legal prerogative of do-not-intubate (DNI). Many investigations have shown during the last decades that despite technological advances, the mortality rate for critically ill oldest-old patients remains high. We know that intensive caring should be able to combine technology and deep humanity, considering that the patients are living the last part of their lives. In addition to the traditional goals of ICU of reducing morbidity and mortality, of maintaining organ functions and restoring health, caring for seriously oldest-old patients should take into account their end-of-life preferences, the advance or proxy directives if available, the prognosis, the communication, their life expectancy, and the impact of comorbidities [9]. In Chap. 9 the decision triage algorithm for COVID-19 proposed by American College of Chest Physicians suggest taking into account the expected risk of mortality based on comorbid conditions and acutely illness using standardised assessment [10]. In this case, the patients may be admitted to an alternative form of caring such as ward with acute care, palliative care setting or even comfort measure only. We think that the risk of mortality assessed by prognostic scores has a meaning different from that of life years to live.

23.5 Conclusion

Many consensuses statements have demonstrated that non-invasive ventilation is a valid alternative therapeutic option out of ICU not only in the sense of palliative and comfort care with a clear significant reduction of the intubation rate in elderly patients although their survival depends on the context in which NIV is applied [11]. Despite better healthcare systems, despite warnings through similar situations and even documented threats, as the COVID-19 pandemic hit, it found us mostly unprepared. It offered to us on a silver tray the fragility of humanity [4]. The effort is to reach guidelines specific for the older patients that physicians can use in hospital clinical pathways in hospital. In this way, we may avoid that SIAARTI makes some specific recommendations to answer to a sudden change in the hospital organisation, to the necessity of resources. Our effort is to continue to work on this project for the future hope that we learn from our mistakes.

References

1. Onder G, Rezza G, Brusaferro S. Case-fatality rate and characteristics of patients dying in relation to COVID-19 in Italy. JAMA. 2020;323(18):1775–6. https://doi.org/10.1001/jama.2020.4683.

2. Vincent J-L, Taccone FS. Understanding pathways to death in patients with COVID-19. Lancet Respir Med. 2020;8(5):430–2. https://doi.org/10.1016/S2213-2600(20)30165-X.
3. http://www.siaarti.it/SiteAssets/News/COVID19%20%20documenti%20SIAARTI/ SIAARTI%20-%20Covid19%20-%20Raccomandazioni%20di%20etica%20clinica.pdf.
4. Cesari M, Proietti M. Geriatric medicine in Italy in the time of Covid-19. J Nutr Health Aging. 2020;3:1–2. https://doi.org/10.1007/s12603-020-1354-z.
5. Aronson L. Age, complexity, and crisis–a prescription for progress in pandemic. N Engl J Med. 2020;383:4–6. https://doi.org/10.1056/NEJMp2006115.
6. Tibullo L, Esquinas AM, Vargas M, et al. Who gets to decide for the older patient with a limited decision-making capacity: a review of surrogacy laws in the European Union. Eur Geriatr Med. 2018;9:759–69. https://doi.org/10.1007/s41999-018-0121-.
7. Legislation.gov.uk. Mental Capacity Act. https://www.legislation.gov.uk/ukpga/2005/9/ contents.
8. Persad G, Wertheimer A, Emanuel EJ. Principles for allocation of scarce medical interventions. Lancet. 2009;373:423–31. https://doi.org/10.1016/S0140-6736(09)60137-9.
9. Vargas N, Tibullo L, Landi E, et al. Caring for critically ill oldest old patients: a clinical review. Aging Clin Exp Res. 2017;29:833–45. https://doi.org/10.1007/s40520-016-0638-y.
10. Maves RC, et al. Triage of scarce critical care resources in COVID-19: an implementation guide for regional allocation: an expert panel report of the task force for mass critical care and the American College of Chest Physicians. Chest. 2020;158(1):212–25.
11. Calvo GS. Definition, criteria and managements of NIV for very old patients with limitation to respiratory care. In: Esquinas AM, Vargas N, editors. Ventilatory support and oxygen therapy in edler, pallaitive and end-of-life care patients. New York: Springer; 2020.

Printed in the United States
by Baker & Taylor Publisher Services